F*CK THE LESSON

Copyright © Fiona McBryde 2024

All rights reserved. No part of this publication may be reproduced, distributed, or transmitted in any form or by any means, including photocopying, recording, or other electronic or mechanical methods, without the prior written permission of the publisher, except in the case of brief quotations embodied in critical reviews and certain other non-commercial uses permitted by copyright law.

(✱) greenhill
https://greenhillpublishing.com.au/

McBryde, Fiona (author)
F*CK THE LESSON
ISBN 978-1-923214-71-2
MEMOIR

Typesetting Calluna Regular 11/18
Cover and book design by Green Hill Publishing

F*CK
THE
LESSON

My wild ride to motherhood
and all the obstacles in between

FIONA McBRYDE

PROLOGUE

THE LAYOUT OF this book is spread across different periods of my life. I have purposely left it this way, as I feel it captures the rawness of what I was going through at the time. It also keeps it authentic, which is important to me. Part 1 was written towards the end of 2017, a time when I felt extremely alone in my journey and, quite frankly, was fed up with the medical industry. I was angry and resentful. I still had my "flair", which is dotted throughout; but when I re-read my book, I can physically feel the pain I was going through when writing Part 1. Part 2 was written towards the end of 2019, after I had received yet another diagnosis, and Part 3 at the end of 2020. Part 4 was written at the end of 2021 and into 2022, and to say that I had been through a lot by this point is an understatement.

I have done my best to keep it raw and honest about how I was feeling. And please remember, this has been *my* experience. In no way am I saying that every single woman has felt the same way, or that I have been failed by any health professional I have seen. I would also like to highlight that I am neither a health professional nor a writer.

The stories in this book are extremely sensitive. I can imagine they will arouse feelings in readers that potentially are unexpected, or that resonate with them on a very intense level. Finally, I would like to say that my journey has shaped me and completely changed me as a person. While it may not have been the road I would have chosen for myself, I have grown exponentially and fully believe that as tough as it has been, it was meant to happen that way. I still don't know what the lesson in all of this is. I'm still learning. But one thing I do know is how very lucky I am, and I never want another woman to feel as alone or desperate or damaged as I have felt throughout my journey.

***Disclaimer:** The names of health professionals mentioned throughout this book have been changed for their own protection. This book is purely my own recollection and personal opinions, and do not reflect those of the health care system or the professionals I have been cared for by. The information throughout this book is not to be used for any form of self-diagnosis or medical purposes – they are purely my own understanding of information provided to me at the time of the event.*

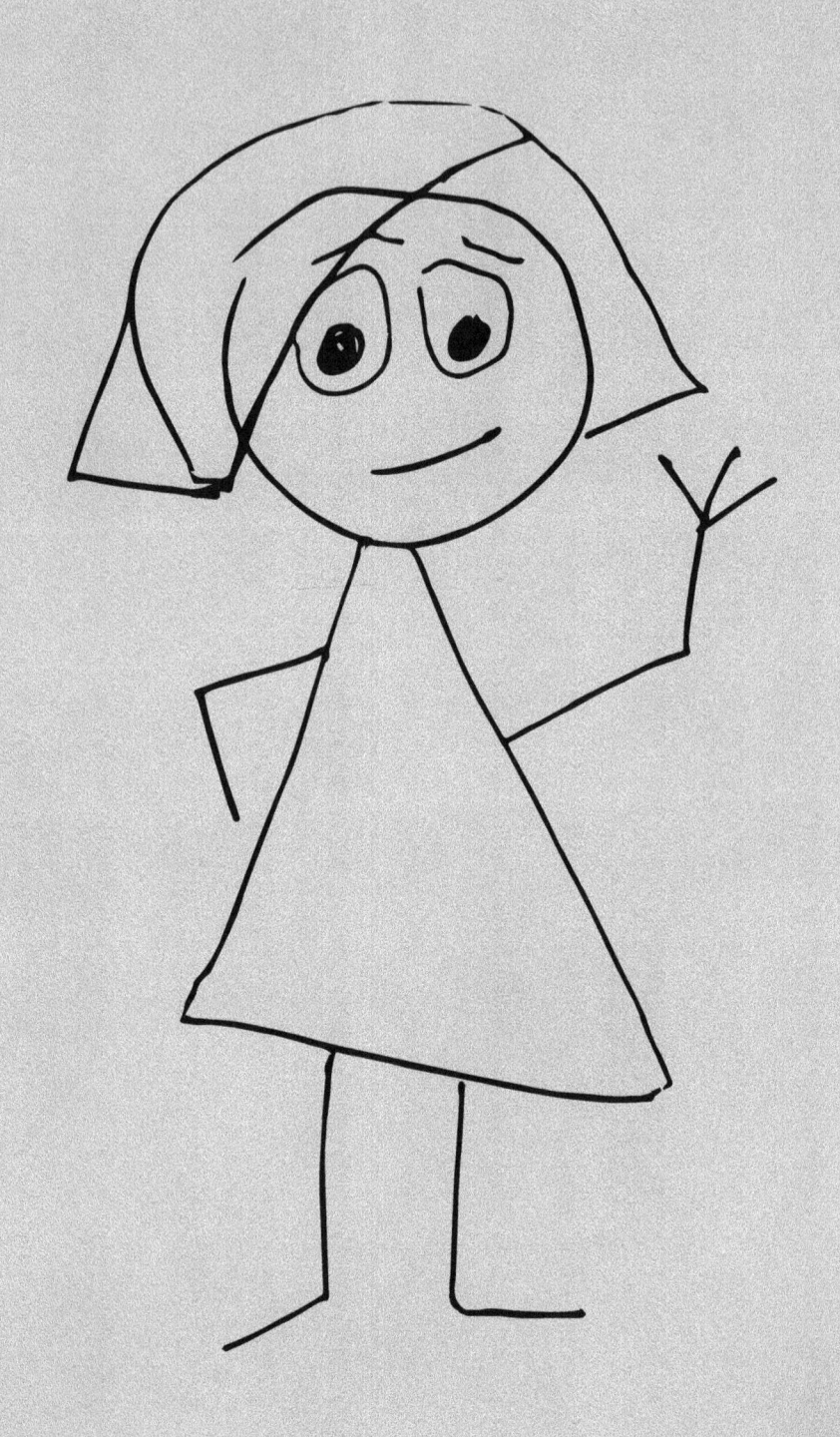

PART 1
A LITTLE ABOUT ME

MY NAME IS Fiona and at the time of writing this, I am 27 years old. I have an amazing husband whose name is Tommy and we have a dog called Zeus who is a pathetic Great Dane cross who thinks he's a Jack Russell. We live in a granny flat on Tommy's parents' property and have done so for the past three years. We love it.

I'm the kind of person who gets straight to the point. Fluffing about in life isn't really my thing. Recently, we've had our third miscarriage in just under two years. I decided to write about our journey because apart from miscarriage still having quite a stigma around it, I enjoy writing and find it therapeutic. Along with that, my coping mechanism is to find the humour in the absolutely crappy things life can throw at us. So why not let everyone in on the journey?

My miscarriages aren't easy thing to talk about. And when I do, I often make jokes about it. I never really saw myself as someone who would have children, to be honest; and so far, it seems that my vision could be a reality. Sorry – just a little dig at myself. I was always your typical teenager, who grew into a twenty-something-year-old saying how much I hated children. I loved my nieces and nephews when they started coming into the world; however, they never fitted in with my hangovers. There is plenty of photographic evidence of me nursing quite a hangover, with one of the children sitting on my lap on a Christmas Day; I always have an awful scowl on my face, while the niece or nephew is thrilled that their Aunty just exists. As I said, I never really saw myself having kids. That was until about three years into my relationship with Tommy, when something in me just clicked.

Tommy had never made a secret about the fact that he wanted to have children, and that he wanted to have them young. My youngest nephew and youngest niece were still quite little when Tommy came onto the scene, and this cemented his idea of having children, especially with me. It took a little longer for me to come to the party, but eventually I was excited at the idea. This was in about 2015. I was 25 and Tommy was 24. At this point I thought that when Tommy was about 40 years old, we'd wake up one day with a bunch of kids and he'd say to me, "You know, we should probably get married, hey." And I was totally fine with that! I was in no rush to get married; I just didn't see it as something that important if you were to have a life with someone. I knew I wanted to be with Tommy forever, and I didn't need a ring or wedding to confirm that.

I was still on contraception at this point, as I had the bar in my arm. However, it had got to the point where I was getting my period every sixteen days, which didn't work for me. My doctor suggested that I stay off contraception for about three months, and let my body get back to normal. We were very careful during this time as I wasn't ready for a pregnancy. After three months I decided to go back on the Pill; more for peace of mind that we wouldn't have an accident. For some reason, though, the Pill was just too random for my body. When I was supposed to get my period, I wouldn't; and when I was taking the Pill religiously every single day, I would end up with my period. So, I decided to come off that after about three months of trying it, and Tommy was fully supportive in this decision.

Tommy and I had discussed having children, but without going into detail, I was grossly taken advantage of in my early teens by someone I trusted, which resulted in me contracting an infection the first time I had sex. Due to the nature of this inappropriate relationship, the infection remained untreated for a significant amount of time. When I finally did receive treatment, I was informed that I may have difficulty conceiving. I had explained that to Tommy and he was very supportive. I think his exact words were: "We'll just see what happens, babe. If we never have kids, that's fine with me." Gotta love him.

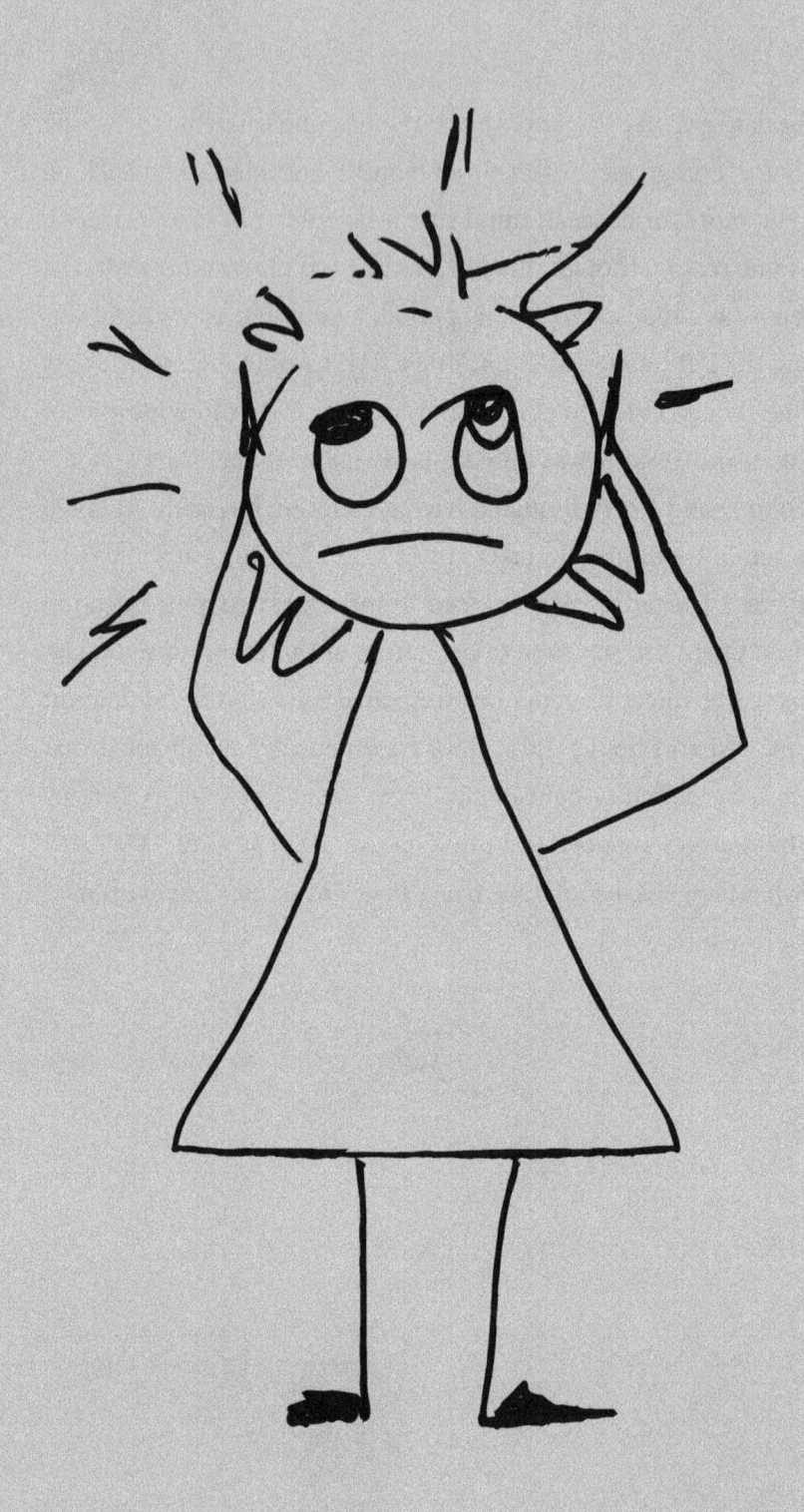

DOUBLE THE TROUBLE

I HAD BEEN off the Pill for one whole cycle, and I got the shock of my life on December 12, 2015, when I had a positive pregnancy test. What the hell! This was supposed to be hard for me.

I can remember the morning vividly. Tommy was still asleep, and I was two days overdue for my period. My boobs were quite sore and I'd been to the toilet four times in an hour. I did the test, not actually thinking it'd be positive; but when I saw that second line start to appear, I thought, Holy shit is this actually happening. I remember sending a photo of the test to my mother, who happens to be a highly renowned midwife in our town, asking her to confirm if I was seeing things or if I was actually pregnant. Needless to say, her response was something along the lines of: "Looks like you'll need a doctor's appointment, lady!"

I'm not sure why, but I was nervous about breaking the news to Tommy. I waited until he woke up, and he was sitting on the couch watching TV when I finally got the courage to tell him. I sat down beside him nervously and said, "Um, babe. So, I did a pregnancy test this morning because I'm a few days late and it was kind of positive…" He looked at me through sleepy eyes and said, "Shit, that was quick!" I felt a sigh of relief. He was totally fine with it.

The following week I went to the doctor and had blood tests done, which confirmed I was approximately five weeks. It was too early for a scan and as we were going away for Christmas, I opted to have one in the first week of the New Year. I can remember feeling seriously pregnant. My boobs were a level of sore I couldn't even explain; it was almost unbearable to even wear a bra. I was visiting the toilet fifty thousand times a day, and my hunger levels were out of control. If this was what pregnancy was like, I totally understood how women put on loads of weight because I could not fill up. I needed a full meal every single hour.

By Week 6, while we were off camping in 10,000-degree heat, I started to feel unwell. Not super sick, just a bit queasy; and if I thought too hard about food, I was really put off by it. I had to have food put in front of me and then I'd be happy to eat it. During the camping trip, I had one episode where I walked up a hill too quickly and everything went white and I almost passed out. That wasn't much fun, so I took it easy for the remainder of the camping trip. Whilst we were camping, Tommy decided he wanted to take me on a date. We didn't do a lot of "dates" as such, so I was excited for a little one-on-one time away from our friends and family for a few hours.

Tommy cooked us a roast chicken, put some VBs in a backpack (for him, obviously), and took me in my brother-in-law's ute to a lookout he'd been wanting to show me, to watch the sun set. Looking back on it, he was acting very strangely. To be honest, I just thought he was drunk, which he probably was a bit! He got lost looking for the track up to the lookout, and at one point he was literally screaming out the window at the sun, "Don't you go down, Sun, ya bastard! Don't you go down!"

Trying to calm him down, I said, "I really appreciate the effort, but we can just find some random hump to watch the sun set if you want? I don't mind." I'm pretty easily pleased and also, I was bloody starving.

After taking another wrong turn, nearly getting bogged, and dinting the bull bar on a giant rock, he finally found the track and absolutely pinned it to the top of this hill, with a few minutes to spare.

As I was walking out over large rocks to get to the lookout, I looked down and saw that someone had been up here cutting trees down. I thought to myself that it was a bit of an extreme place to come and get firewood; but I was also too hungry to care, so made myself comfortable and started hooking into the roast chicken while Tommy followed behind me. Little did I know, Tommy and my brother-in-law had been up here earlier that day cutting trees down so we could have a perfect view of the sunset. Tommy sat down beside me and cracked open a VB. Classy. I was chowing down on the chicken he'd cooked earlier, and he asked me if I was excited for next year. Through a full mouth I said yes, but that it was going to be a big year for sure. I was due on August 20th, which also happened to be my grandfather's birthday. He had passed away before I was born, but I felt it was a good omen. Our conversation went something like this:

Me: "Yeah, of course I'm excited. It will be a big year, though. We've got a bit to get in order between now and August, that's for sure. Are you excited for next year?"

Tommy: "Yeah, I am. But there's one thing I'm not happy with and I really want it to change."

I can remember this moment vividly. Had he brought me up on this nice date, to this nice hill, with a nice meal, just to pick a fight with me? *Okay, mate, let's do this,* I thought.

Me: "Yeah, righto. And what's that?" This was said in a very icy tone. I was ready for an argument.

Tommy: "I want to start the new year with you as my wife-to-be..." he said, pulling a box out of his backpack.

I dived over and tackled him, cry-screaming, "What the fuck is wrong with you?" I couldn't believe it. I had not seen that coming at all! It now totally made sense that he had been so stressed trying to find the track. He couldn't believe I hadn't figured it out, but I spend most of my life in my own little world and this was no different. I honestly had no clue. Obviously, I said yes, and once the sun went down, we went back to camp to celebrate not only the New Year but our engagement.

We headed home on New Year's Day and my first scan was booked for mid-January. Unfortunately, Tommy couldn't make it, so I took my mum with me. Having never had this type of scan before, I couldn't really see what we were looking for. I could see a few things going on, but as she took pictures of my uterus the girl's only words were, "Okay, I can see a couple of things going on here." I can remember thinking, *Oh God, don't say a couple, imagine if it was twins.* Nothing was really explained to me during the scan, and the results were sent to my doctor. I had an appointment for the following afternoon.

My normal doctor wasn't available, so I had a substitute, who was very nice. She reviewed the scan report and said, "So it's twins! Identical, actually." I stared at her blankly and said, "Pardon?" she repeated herself. I couldn't believe it. How on earth was I going to tell Tommy? My mother's house was right around the corner from the doctor's office, so after my appointment I sped around there, stormed up the stairs and waved the report at her saying, "Its twins!"

She looked at me and laughed and said, "Well, I did think there were two in there yesterday but scans aren't really my area of expertise." She was in hysterics. I hadn't even realised that we had twins in the family. It turns out my grandfather had twin brothers. Great. For someone who never saw herself with kids, this was all becoming a bit overwhelming, but Mum was so excited.

Meanwhile, I was thinking, *This is my karma for all those years of saying I'd never have children.* I drove home trying to think of how to break the news to Tommy. When I got there, Tommy came racing out of the house to greet me. I looked at him and said, "Yeah, everything is fine. Just come inside for a sec." I think he could tell I was seriously anxious because his face dropped, and he stood in the doorway trying to read me.

"What happened?" he asked.

"Okay, there's no other way to say this. It's twins." My eyes were as big as saucers as I delivered the news. I was waiting for him to flip out.

It took him a second, but he burst out laughing and said, "Well shit, I didn't spill any then, did I!"

I instantly relaxed and laughed at his response, but it was the perfect answer. I pulled the report out and showed him, and he was over the moon. Thank God. Our heads were spinning with happiness, excitement and a little anxiety; but overall, we were absolutely stoked. The doctor had ordered me a scan for the following week as, because of the size of the babies, they were only able to get one heartbeat, which was apparently normal. The other baby was measuring slightly smaller, so I was to return the following week for another scan to make sure we had both heartbeats.

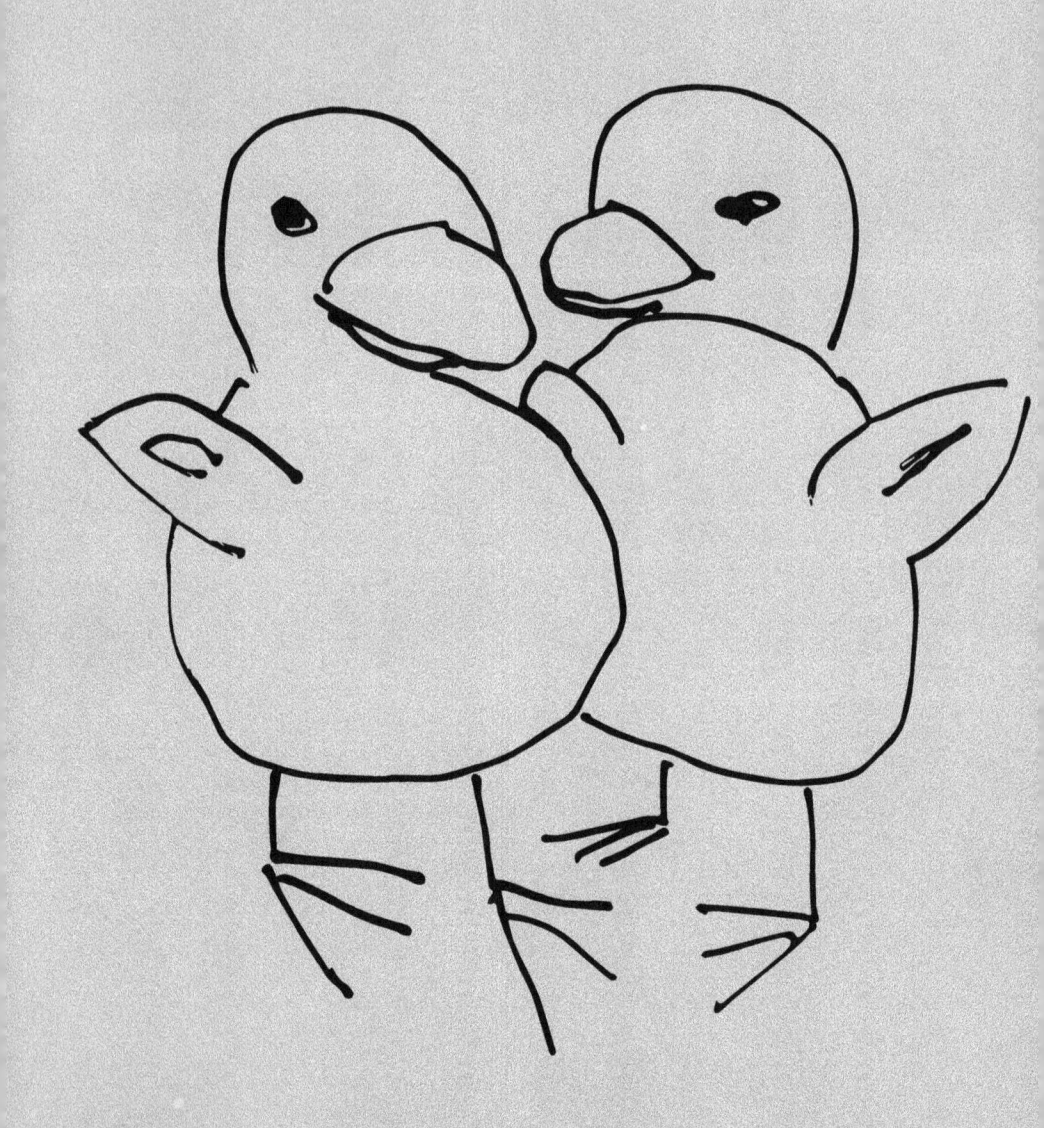

WHEN YOU KNOW, YOU KNOW

THE NEXT SCAN was performed on January 21st, 2016. It was a horrible day. Unfortunately, Tommy was again unable to make it to the scan, so I took my mother. I was dreading it. A part of me knew it was going to be bad news. I felt that my boobs had stopped being sore, and my appetite didn't seem as intense. Aside from having this gut feeling that things weren't right, the experience with the sonographer was terrible. After a few moments into the ultrasound, the young woman obviously knew there was a problem. She turned the screen off so I couldn't see anything for myself, and she didn't say anything throughout the entire scan.

When I asked her what was going on, she said, "Our screens have been playing up, so I've had to turn it off." I tried to ask her what she could see, and she just kept saying, "A report will be sent to your doctor."

My advice to any sonographers out there is: DO NOT DO THIS. This was the worst possible thing anyone could do to an expectant mother. Let her see for herself what is happening. I understand it is not necessarily your job to say, "I'm not getting a heartbeat for either of the babies, and they haven't grown since the last scan." But do not shut the poor mother out from being able to see things herself. We're not stupid, and chances are we already know something is wrong; so don't be so insensitive as to shut us off from our own damn uterus!

Still not having been told what they had or hadn't seen, I was asked to wait in the waiting room while they called my doctor. It was appalling. My anxiety was through the roof and my mind was racing like crazy. Of course, I knew it was bad news; it was 4.30pm and they were desperately trying to contact my doctor. I was so thankful that Mum was with me for this, as I had started to spiral. She kept telling me to remain positive, which I'm sure was for her own reassurance as well.

Finally, the report had been sent and one of the other office ladies came over to me and said, "We've called your doctor and she's waiting for you at her practice. Please head straight there now and she'll explain the results."

Gee, thanks, love. But I already know what's happening and if the stupid lady doing my ultrasound had left the screen on for me to see for myself, I wouldn't be working myself up so much right now!

We got to my GP, who is the most beautiful woman I have ever had the pleasure of dealing with. She used to work with my mother as well, so I think having to deliver the news to both of us was even harder for her. Now, I'm not a typical person when it comes to receiving bad news. I need it direct, I need to know the next step, and it all needs to be in black and white. I really struggle with people trying to get all emotional about it. Just give me this shit straight so I can process it. I remember my doctor explaining what had happened. She said that the scan had shown no heartbeats or growth in either foetus and I had had a miscarriage.

"Okay, so what happens next?" I asked matter-of-factly.

"Fiona, I don't think you're understanding what I'm telling you. Take a moment to take it in. Unfortunately, you've had a miscarriage and there is no cardiac activity in either foetus," she said ever so sweetly.

Looking back, I regret being as rude as I was. "No. I understand that they're gone, but what happens next? How do we get them out? What is the next step?"

I looked at my mother. She had tears in her eyes for me, and my doctor passed her a tissue.

Finally, I got the explanation of what happened next, and I allowed myself to cry. My doctor told me to take the weekend to think about whether I wanted to wait for the sac to come out naturally, which could take weeks, or have medical intervention by way of using Misoprostol or having a curette.

Mum drove me back to her place, where I desperately tried to call Tommy but couldn't get him on the phone. When he eventually called me back, trying to get the words out was the hardest thing I've ever had to do.

"I lost them…" I cried down the phone. "I'm so sorry. I'm so sorry," I kept saying.

Tommy, being the beautiful human that he is, just said, "Babe, don't be sorry. It's okay. Are you okay? Do you want me to come and pick you up? I'm so sorry I'm not there with you."

I felt awful. Literally the week before that, Tommy had crawled into bed and kissed my stomach saying, "Just saying good night to the twins." It had made my heart explode, and now it was in a million pieces from telling him I'd lost them.

Anyone who has ever had a miscarriage knows that nothing anyone can say or do for you will make you feel better. It's shit. That feeling of loss and complete emptiness is unforgettable. And the sadness of everyone else around you is completely harrowing. I don't think I've ever felt as broken as I did that day. Mum dropped me home and Tommy met me with a massive hug. He helped me inside to bed, where I lay crying for such a long time. I couldn't believe this had happened. How? No one in my family had ever had a miscarriage. My grandmother was one of sixteen, my mum one of six, I was one of three, and my two older sisters had had two and three children respectively. Why me? Being a twin pregnancy, the risk of miscarriage is always higher than for a singular. But as you can imagine, this information didn't help me feel better at all.

Over the weekend, we made the decision that we would seek medical intervention by Misoprostol to get them out. I didn't want to wait weeks and I hadn't experienced any spotting, so I wanted to get this over with. The following Monday I went back to my GP, who unfortunately was away, so I had to get the referral to the hospital from another doctor. She called ahead for me and let the hospital know I was on my way.

I was admitted to ED, where they took bloods and did a scan. One of the nurses who was looking after me asked some questions, and after I told her it was a twin pregnancy she asked if they were identical or unidentical. When I told her they were identical her response, I kid you not, was: "Oh, they're the common ones; you don't want them anyway. It's unidentical you want – they're unique!" I wasn't really sure what to do with this information. I think I just stared blankly at her for a moment and turned back to the screen. What a stupid thing to say.

Nothing was easy in the withdrawal process of this failed pregnancy. Because it was a twin pregnancy, my blood levels had more than quadrupled; and even though the hospital had their own scan along with the report from the week before, confirming no cardiac activity in either foetus, I was sent home. I was told to come back in a week because my bloods were too high for them to do anything. When the on-call doctor in ED told me there was nothing they could do, I completely broke down. I just wanted this to all be over. I had mentally prepared myself to have the Misoprostol, only to be told I had to wait another week. I was shattered!

Thankfully, the following day was a public holiday, so I had a day to regather myself before going back to work for another week. Did I mention I'm a complaints officer for an electricity company? Let me just say, while you're going through this, and customers want to complain about the fact that they lost power during a storm for an hour and that in this day and age power loss during storms shouldn't happen, it takes all your strength not to tell them where to shove it. Trust me.

Thankfully, Monday the 1st of February finally rolled around. As my mother worked at this hospital, she had arranged for one of the doctors on the maternity ward to insert the Misoprostol. Being the beautiful woman my mother is, she had also informed the doctor not to faff about with me and to deliver any advice or what l should expect in black and white terms. Bless her. Additional bloods were taken prior to seeing the doctor, to ensure that my HCG levels had indeed fallen since the week before. Part of me was so hopeful that some sort of miracle had occurred and the babies were alive. Of course, that was not the case.

Now, l find humour in some pretty sick situations. By no means was any of this funny at the time, but looking back on it l can see there was one moment that l find pretty hilarious. I was given my own room and my bloods came back confirming a significant drop in HCG levels from the week before. Awesome – green light. The doctor came in and apologised for my loss and explained what was going to happen. Tommy sat beside me listening intently to what was going to follow. The doctor explained there were two tablets; she would insert the first one just underneath my cervix and within a few hours it would begin to dilate. The second tablet I was to insert myself the following day at the same time. Okay, l could do this.

Here we go. The doctor put her gloves on and felt around inside me. After having a few internal scans and pap smears in the past, this didn't really faze me. She looked me dead in the eyes and said, "Can you feel me touching your cervix there?" l don't deal with eye contact very well at the best of times, but while you've got your hand up in my grill, poking my cervix, and you're asking if l can feel it… well, this was all a bit too much. I almost lost my shit laughing. I nodded and looked over at Tommy, who looked like a deer caught in headlights as he watched this woman with her hand inside me. I just had to have a bit of a giggle to myself. She pulled her fingers out and put the tablet back in. I thanked her for her help, and we were off on our merry way.

By about 8pm I had started to bleed. I decided to go to bed because I didn't really want to deal with it by this point. On Tuesday 2nd February, 2016, at approximately 6.00am I went to the toilet and looked down. Just in time, I was able to grab a handful of toilet paper and catch the sac before it fell in the toilet. I had just passed my babies. The sac was approximately 5cm long and about 2cm wide. I didn't inspect it too much as I found it all a bit too confronting. I wrapped them up in toilet paper and placed them in a small box my mum had brought me. I went back to bed and cuddled up to Tommy and cried. I felt numb. It felt like I was living in slow motion or watching a movie of my life. How could this possibly be real life? Who starts their day by catching a sac of their dead babies? It was so traumatic, something no one should ever have to deal with.

That day Mum took me to a nursery to buy a nice fruit tree to plant above where I would bury my babies. I thought it was a good idea, and looking back on it I am eternally grateful she dragged me out of the house to do this. We bought a peach tree. And to go with it, we bought a little duckling ornament that had a bigger duck with his wing holding on to a smaller duck cuddling into him. It was perfect. I got home that afternoon and planted my babies in a nice big pot on my front verandah, with the peach tree on top and the duckling ornament facing the doorway of the house. It made me so happy that every single day as I walked out of the house, I would be greeted by my peach tree.

Prior to having my own miscarriage, I could never really understand what people go through. Until you have one, you cannot understand or wrap your head around what that person must be going through. As I said earlier, nothing anyone says and no advice they try to give will make you feel any better. The hardest pill to swallow is the shitty advice people feel the need to give you after you've had a miscarriage. Seriously, things like: "it just wasn't meant to be"; "it's all about your frame of mind, body and soul; if it's right then it will all work out"; "you really just need to concentrate on yourself and reassess your diet; make sure you're eating well, taking folic acid and exercising regularly"; "maybe it was a blessing in disguise? ... you guys maybe just weren't ready for kids, and it was your body's way of helping you out"; "at least it was early". A little piece of advice to anyone who knows someone that has a miscarriage. Don't say any of this shit. Just sit there, tell them you're sorry for their loss and hand them a big old glass of wine. You might think these are helpful, spiritual things to say, but they're not. Just agree that it is shit and unfair and it sucks that it happened and refill their goddamn glass.

About a fortnight after I had passed the sac, I had been scheduled for another scan to make sure everything had come out. The lady I saw was lovely, and she herself had suffered a miscarriage so she completely understood the importance of letting me see my own uterus. I'll never forget her words after she brought up a clear view of my empty uterus. "You did a beautiful job, darling," she said. Such a simple sentence and meant with such empathy. I remember walking out of that scan, making it to my car and crying my eyes out. It was such a lovely thing to say, but I felt that her words insinuated I had given birth. As if I'd done a fantastic job delivering a lifeless sac. Go me. I tried to take it the way she meant it, but her empathy and genuine hurt for me broke my heart. I didn't feel like I deserved that sort of respect. I hadn't gone through labour like mothers do. Yes, I had suffered through physical pain, and continued to suffer through emotional pain, but I didn't feel worthy of her kind words.

My first miscarriage, I will admit, will always be my most painful both physically and emotionally. I still get upset at the thought of losing my twins. I still hurt on a daily basis thinking of my beautiful babies, even if they were common, identical twins, who would be over twelve months old now and would have seriously cheeky personalities. Their due date of August 20th has now passed me by more than once, and I've spent each time in tears. Those little devils (and I can quite confidently say they would be little devils) would have driven me crazy, made me laugh, and kept me on my toes. But I would have loved those babies so damn hard, and our house would have been filled with laughter, singing and a family of four who got a serious case of hangry every few hours. It would have been a riot; Tommy and I would have loved it.

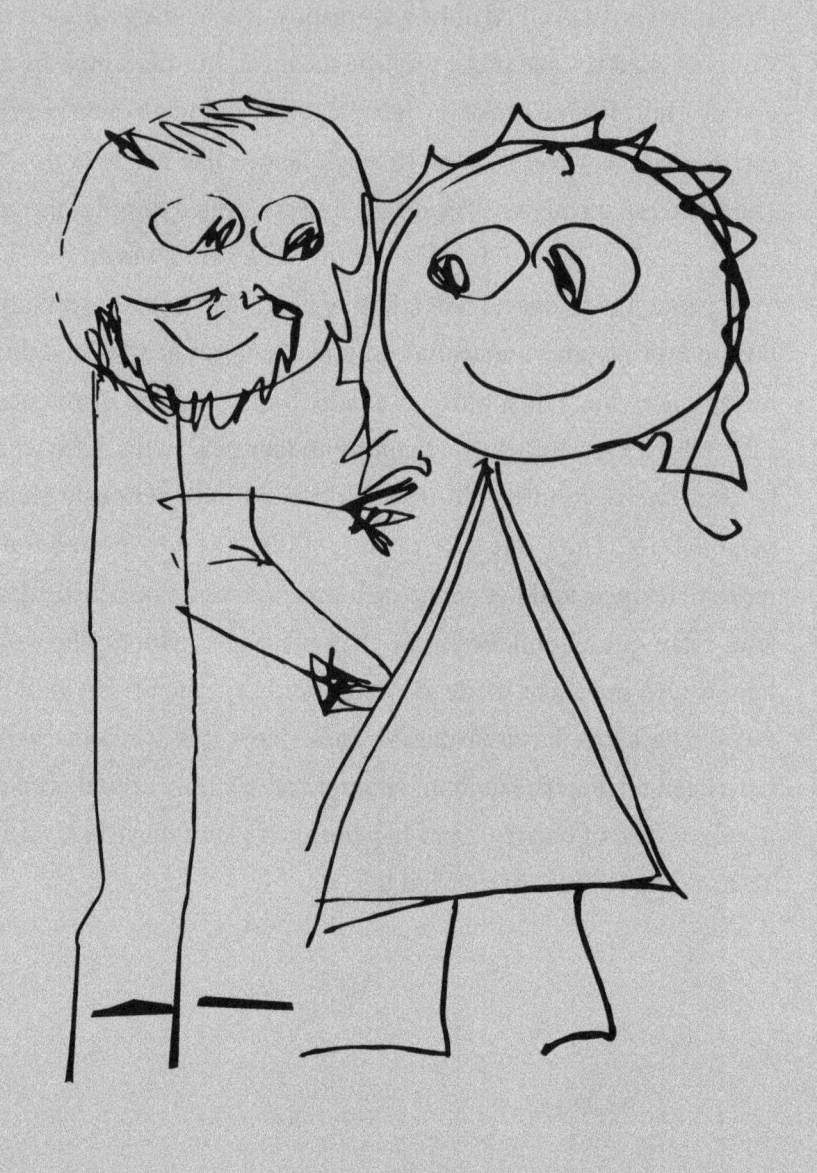

IT'S NOT ALL DOOM AND GLOOM

FOR A FEW months after I miscarried the twins, Tommy and I tried to fall pregnant again. Unfortunately, I think we tried too hard, and it just wasn't meant to be. I went back on the Pill in May 2016 as we had set the date for our wedding the following year in April, and I didn't want to be a big pregnant lady at the wedding. Not that there is anything wrong with being pregnant at your wedding, I just didn't want that for myself.

Mostly, the rest of 2016 was a great year. We went on plenty of camping trips with family and friends, and purchased our first camper trailer which we were pretty excited about. Our wedding date was fast approaching, and we'd picked Canada for our honeymoon destination. There was so much to look forward to! From May to November 2016, I remained on the Pill and I battled with the fact that my period was inconsistent, and I would never get it when I was supposed to. By November, I was over it so I came off the Pill again. I figured if I fell pregnant between then and the wedding, my dress would still fit and I'd be able to hide it, or it would be time to announce it anyway.

December and January came and went, and I still got my period. In February, I decided to make sure I was definitely ovulating and opted to use ovulation sticks, to make sure I was ovulating when I thought I was. I got the positive ovulation test and Tommy and I had sex for the next few days to give us the best possible chance of falling pregnant. On March 10th 2017, I got my period and I was devastated. I remember crying my eyes out to my mother, explaining that we had been trying to get pregnant for a few months and it just wasn't happening. Why? Why wasn't it happening? I was so angry and frustrated with my body. Just do your damn job and fall pregnant! Mum felt really sad for me and reminded me I was getting married in less than a month and then going on the holiday of a lifetime. She encouraged me to relax and enjoy our wedding and honeymoon, and deal with baby stuff after the wedding. It was great advice.

Two weeks before our wedding we traded in our camper trailer and purchased a brand spanking new caravan. We're crazy, I know! But we were both so excited to get it that we drove to Mackay and stayed in a caravan park to test it out. To celebrate, we got a heap of drinks and nibblies and Tommy played barman for the evening. I don't remember much but Tommy informs me we had a great time. I woke up in what I thought was the early hours of the morning, but really it was about 9.00pm. I felt like I was going to throw up. Being naked, I grabbed the closest thing to me which was Tommy's t-shirt, threw it on, and ran across the caravan park to the toilets to be sick.

In my head, the shirt covered my dignity and the patrons in the park were none the wiser to the fact I had no underwear on. According to Tommy, this was not the case. He informed me the next morning that we were parked directly under a floodlight and the entire park copped a view of my white backside as I ran across the park to the toilets. Whoops! Needless to say, I was one sick human driving home the next day.

Before long, our wedding day had arrived. I was due to get my period the day after our wedding, and my boobs were tender in the week leading up to the wedding which was a good indication my period was on its way. We started the day off with wine and finished it with vodka. It was, hands down, the greatest day of my life. Getting to marry my best friend and party with our closest family and friends was seriously awesome. I was a little worse for wear the following morning, and discreetly threw up in the toilets before and after breakfast. Cute, I know.

We were due to fly out that evening, so it was a mad rush to pack up, get home and get back to the airport in time for our flight. I remember feeling very overwhelmed by everyone's love this day. I basically had a lump in my throat the entire day, and saying thank you/goodbye to people was very emotional for me. I figured it was because my period was due, so I was a bit more fragile than normal. We made our flight and went straight to bed, as we had an early flight to Canada the following morning.

We arrived in Calgary, Canada, on Monday 10th April local time, and drove to Banff where we were booked to stay for a few days. It was a long-ass trip but we made it. It was early evening when we got to Banff so we quickly freshened up and headed to a pub for dinner. We both had a few drinks, swung past a pharmacy on the way home to get some drowsy antihistamines, and went home. I still didn't have my period; but I figured that with the long flight and stress of the wedding, maybe my body was confused and I'd get it in a few days. I wasn't really concerned.

We woke the following morning at about 8:30am, a casual 14 hours after crawling into bed. Tommy has a tendency to get pretty weird in his sleep when he is overtired, and this was no exception. I woke up during the night to see Tommy stumbling out of bed and trying to go out of the front door into the hallway, looking for the toilet. After I yelled at him, he angrily responded, "I need to wee!" He then proceeded to walk straight into a wall, told the wall to fuck off, then felt his way along it to safely find the right place to wee. The poor guy had absolutely no idea where he was, and he didn't really have much recollection of the incident the following morning. We spent the day planning our stay in Banff and organising gear for hire to go snowboarding.

The following morning, we woke early for a day on the slopes. We headed to a nearby ski area called Sunshine Village, and having not boarded for three years we were keen to see if we could remember how to do it. Tommy was all over it, but I was a bit wobbly. We had a great instructor who was a fellow Aussie, and had done about four seasons at Sunshine Village. By the end of our two-hour lesson, we were both thrilled with our progress. Tommy of course was top of the class and hungry for more. I was just hungry. After lunch we had another two-hour lesson with the same instructor, who told us it was completely normal to stiffen up and become exhausted.

After about an hour into our second lesson, I decided to call it a day. The chairlifts were making me feel sick and I knew I needed to rest. I waited for Tommy to finish his lesson and when he finally came to meet me, we got back in the gondola to head down the mountain to the car park. I was feeling particularly sick in the gondola on the way down, and the motion of it just wasn't agreeing with me at all. I'm no stranger to motion sickness, but this was different. On the way home we decided to grab a pregnancy test just to check. I certainly didn't feel pregnant, but my period was now three days late and wasn't showing any signs of arriving.

We got back to the room and I went straight to the toilet. Not expecting it to be positive, I jumped in the shower while I waited for the stick to show the result. When I got out of the shower and saw those two lines showing a positive pregnancy test, I couldn't believe it. I felt completely different to last time, so how in the world was it positive? I mean, I had tender boobs, but I always got those around my period. I was hungry, but I'm a pretty hungry human in general.

I walked out of the bathroom and said to Tommy blankly, "So, it's positive... I'm pregnant."

His face lit up and he said, "Really? That's awesome!" He was stoked. A little marshmallow was on its way. I on the other hand, felt uneasy.

The following three weeks went by way too quickly. We had a blast in Canada, and got to experience the most amazing things like snowmobiling and dog sledding. We also met the Canadian version of Tommy and Fiona, and we remain in contact with them today. We hope one day to get back to visit them.

We arrived home on April 30th 2017. Thankfully, Monday 1st May was a public holiday, so we had one more day before going back to work. I wanted to talk to my mother about being pregnant. Something about it just didn't feel right, and as positive as I was trying to be, I kept saying to Tommy that I didn't feel pregnant, and I had to keep reminding myself that I was. I had all the right symptoms – hunger, growing boobs, slight nausea – but something was just "off".

I was standing in my mother's bathroom and I said to her, "So, I'm pregnant. But before you get excited, I don't feel pregnant, so I'm trying not to get my hopes up."

I could see the worry in her eyes, but she did her best to reassure me and told me that she was never sick and only had sore boobs as a symptom of pregnancy. I had wanted to wait until I was at least eight weeks pregnant before going for a scan. Unfortunately, my body had other plans.

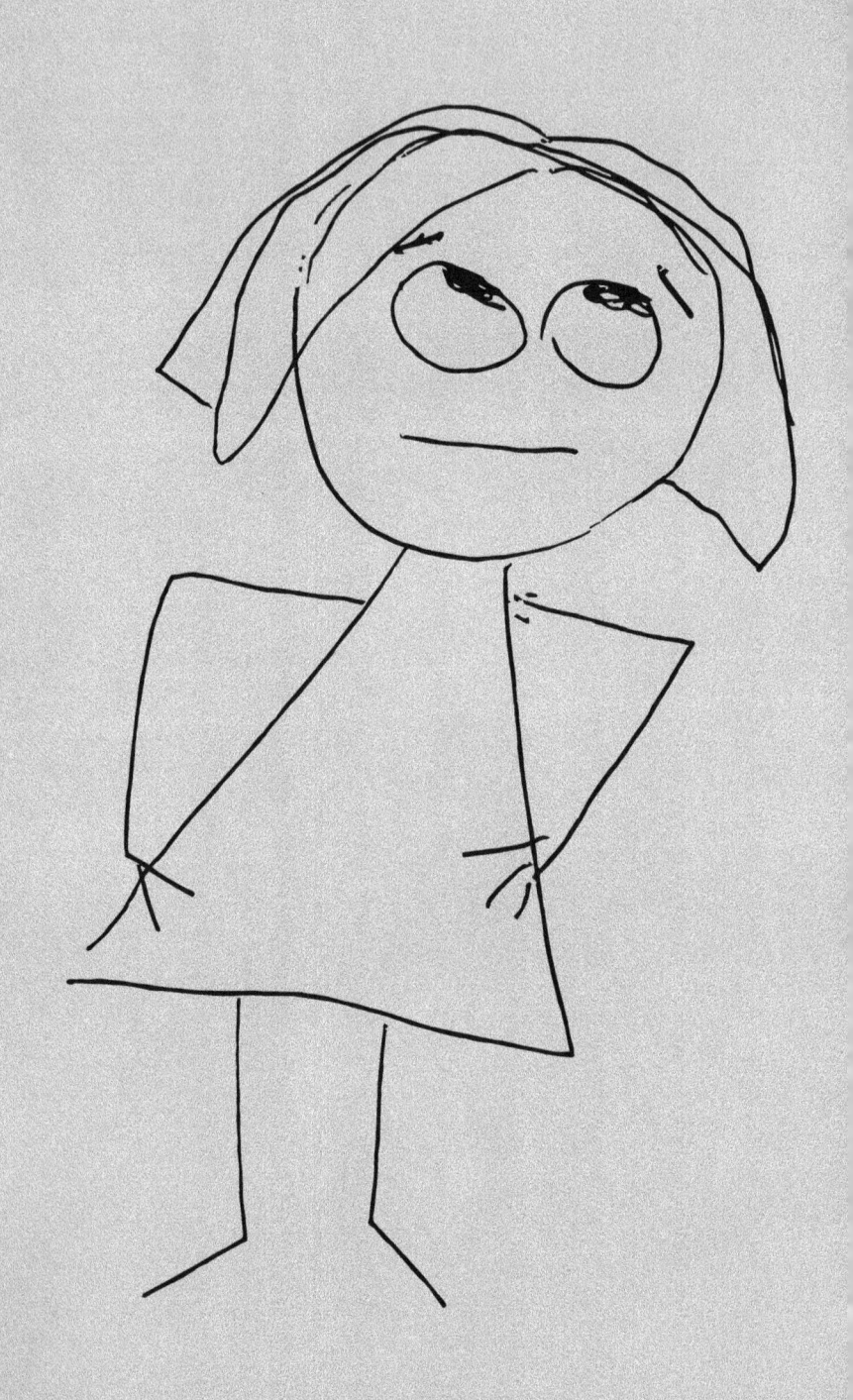

HERE WE GO AGAIN

ON THE EVENING of Wednesday 3rd May, I had no pain, but I could feel warmth in my underwear. I went to the toilet and saw quite a lot of deep red blood. Autopilot kicked in and a familiar sensation of pure numbness started to settle over me. After putting a pad in my underwear, I rang Mum and explained calmly what had happened. She had her own private midwifery practice by this point, and her partner arranged for me to have a scan the following day, and I had bloods taken earlier that morning.

Our scan was at about 2.00pm and Tommy was able to come with me. I can remember standing outside the sonographers, and I said to Tommy, "I bet you any money the bloods will be bang on for how far we are, but the scan will be bad news." He encouraged me to remain positive and just wait and see. Shortly before the scan, Mum texted me the results of the bloods, and they were in perfect range for someone who was about seven weeks pregnant. My gut feeling was proving to be right.

We got into the scan, and I told the girl that I'd had some bleeding and to please not turn the monitor off because this was my second pregnancy and I wanted to see things for myself. Thankfully, she obliged. A clear picture of my uterus came into view, and the girl didn't need to say anything. I could see for myself – it was completely empty. From all accounts there was nothing there to see. She quietly apologised and said she needed to take some photos of my uterus. I wasn't surprised. I knew that was how it was going to play out.

I remember thinking that my uterus looked different to last time. It was as if there was snow across the screen in the shape of grape bunches. I didn't think anything of it, texted my mother to let her know the outcome, and went home. I can't remember crying much at this point. I think I'd already come to terms with the fact that I didn't feel pregnant, so I didn't feel like I'd actually lost anything this time. It was still sad, but it didn't feel as emotionally painful.

As my referring midwife, the report had been sent to my mother's business partner. It wasn't good news. Mum rang me and tried to explain the results of the scan.

"So, the scan has shown your uterus to have the appearance of GTD, which stands for gestational trophoblastic disease. It doesn't mean you have it; it just means that we'll need to organise for you to come up to the hospital and book you in for a curette if you don't pass it naturally, because it does have the potential to become cancerous."

I'm sure she explained more, but all I remember hearing is "cancerous" and I immediately panicked. I do have a bit of a tendency for going from zero to one hundred in a hypochondriac sense, so I'd pretty much diagnosed myself with cancer at this point. Stupid, I know. I hung up the phone, waited for Tommy to come home, and asked him to just call Mum so she could explain; otherwise I would freak him out. He tried to get it out of me, and all I could blurt out through hysterical crying was the dreaded 'c' word. So he called Mum and got the actual diagnosis, which really wasn't bad at all.

I went up to the hospital on the Friday and was given a specimen cup in case I passed any tissue over the weekend; otherwise I was booked in for surgery the following Monday. To get our minds off the fact we'd only just come back from an amazing holiday to shit-house news, we decided to take the caravan out for the weekend with my sisters and their families. It was a great weekend. I had a good time riding motorbikes and spending time with my nieces and nephews, whom I had seriously missed while we were away. On the Sunday morning I passed what looked like a small grape bunch, and managed to capture it in the specimen cup. On the way back into town from camping, I rang Mum to let her know, and she organised for me to come up to the hospital to be examined. The specimen was taken away for testing and the on-call doctor felt my cervix and confirmed it was closed, so was confident I had passed it. Great! No surgery. Phew. Because my uterus had shown the appearance of GTD, I was given four blood request forms to have a week apart for the next four weeks, to make sure my beta HCG levels were reducing. Anything was better than surgery.

I decided not to go to work the following week. It had been traumatic with the cancer scare and I needed some time to get over it. By Tuesday morning the 9th of May, I woke up feeling less than ordinary.

I had an awful headache, was having serious waves of intense period pain and I couldn't work out why. I lay on the couch for a few hours and wasn't really getting much bleeding, but I decided to go in to Mum and see what she thought I should do. While I was there, I went to the toilet and passed what I thought was a sizeable clot.

My poor mother put gloves on and fished it out of the toilet to get a closer look at it and, bless her, said, "I've seen bigger. The positive thing here is it's better out than in."

I decided to head home to a heat pack and bed because I was just honestly feeling so rough. While at home, I went to the toilet again and passed an even bigger clot. I thought it was huge. It would have been easily 8cm long and about 3cm wide. Massive to me. Mum encouraged me to see my beautiful GP the following day, to maybe get another scan just to make sure everything was gone.

I woke up feeling much better and had stopped bleeding as heavily; just some light spotting. I went to my GP, and she ordered me a scan which I was able to have the same day. I went up to the hospital radiology for this scan and was met by a young girl who appeared to recognise me. She looked familiar, but I honestly was in no mood to try and work out how we knew each other, and she didn't have a name tag on, so I just let her do her thing. Every time I had had an ultrasound, no matter the amount of water I did or didn't drink, my bladder was always too full, and we had to go to an internal scan. Which, quite honestly, I preferred because it was a better view. This lovely young girl informed me to just go with an empty bladder because most sonographers prefer to do internal anyway. Good to know. I didn't want to see the screen for this scan because I didn't care. I knew there wasn't a baby in there, so what was there to see?

I had explained to the girl about my trauma from the twin pregnancy where the girl turned the monitor off and wouldn't tell me anything. She was horrified that someone would do that, and made sure I was well informed about my uterus this time.

She said to me, "When are you seeing your doctor again, Fiona?" I told her I had an appointment at 9.00am for the following morning. She advised, "Okay, that's great. Make sure you go because there is still some tissue in your uterus, so you'll need to have that removed. I'll get this report sent over to your doctor as soon as possible so it's there for her in the morning. Okay?"

ARE YOU SERIOUS?! I've gone through the pain of miscarrying, passed what I felt was a massive amount of tissue, been told my cervix is closed, and now I'm going to have to have surgery anyway. Sorry for the language, but this right here, for me, was a major "fuck my life" moment.

I called my mother and told her what the sonographer had said. She provided me with the name of a female obstetrician and said to ask my GP to refer me to her for the operation. This was bullshit. I showed up to my GP and she delivered the news.

"Yeah, yeah, I know. Can you please refer me to Dr A*? Once the referral is sent through, I'll call and make an appointment." I realise that I had been quite rude to my GP, and as I said, she is the most beautiful and loving woman; but I unfortunately am a shitty recipient of this sort of kindness when I'm in the middle of a traumatic life event. It's something I'm working on.

The referral was faxed through, and I decided to go and get myself some comfort food. I had planned to call Dr A's office after I had eaten, so I went to my sister's place (she lived near the hospital) to eat my brunch. Whilst driving to my sister's place, I received a phone call from Dr A's office and was asked to come up for an appointment at 12:30pm. That was quick! I think it was at this moment that I realised the seriousness of the situation, and how just having your uterus show the appearance of GTD could end badly.

I walked into my sister's house. She was in the middle of a teleconference so she just gave a caring wave and smile. I sat down at the table and her husband said, "How you going, Fi?" Under normal circumstances, a completely harmless question. For this point in time, heartbreaking. I burst into tears and ran to the bathroom. I sat on the toilet crying my eyes out.

Why was this happening to me? I'm a good person and I don't deserve this shit. Was this punishment for something? Seriously, what had I done in life to cop such a harsh deal? My sister opened the door with tears in her eyes. She was in pain for me and seeing me so distraught hurt her as well.

"What did the doctor say?"

Through sloppy tears and snot bubbles, I managed to get out that I'd been referred to the obstetrician and had to be there by 12.30 pm. This was all happening so fast. Mum was unfortunately out of town, and Tommy was working approximately 50 minutes south of our hometown, so he wouldn't be able to make it back for the appointment. Thankfully, my sister agreed to come with me.

Dr A was lovely. She was very matter-of-fact, which I needed by that point, and explained to me how the curette was going to work. She asked a series of normal questions for when one has had a miscarriage: "Did you drink alcohol? Take drugs? Any other medication?" And she proceeded to tell me that more often than not it was just a chromosomal abnormality. Based on my scans, there was also the concern that it might be a molar pregnancy. She tried to explain this to me but to be honest, it was all going in one ear and out the other. I figured I could google it later and freak myself out more, just like most people who google medical things. She asked me when I'd last eaten and I told her about 10:30am. She told me to fast from here on in and to be back at the hospital by 3.30pm, ready for the surgery shortly after 5.00pm when she'd finished her practice for the day. What? I was getting surgery today? She sent me off for more bloods before surgery and said, "See you later."

Shit! I rang Tommy and informed him that I needed to be back at the hospital by 3.30pm. He told me he'd be back in time and would pack an overnight bag for me just in case, and would meet me at the hospital. We lived about 40 minutes north of the hospital so for me to go home and come back in time was near impossible.

I went back to my sister's house and showered in preparation for the surgery. The time seemed to come around ridiculously quickly, and I went back up to the hospital to pay and get admitted. I was given the attractive surgery gown, the nurse put those tight socks on my legs, and I waited. I was nervous. The last time I'd gone under anaesthetic I was 14 and had a pin put in my right wrist. When I came out of surgery I was vomiting and hallucinating. Not a fun time at all. I didn't want that to happen again.

Tommy finally arrived, before I met with the anaesthetist. We went in a little room to chat. He was the nicest man. His name was

Dominic* and he explained what his role in my operation was. He said to me, "Normally, when it's a case of elective surgery my costs would go outside the Medicare and your health fund gap. In this case, I know you don't want to be here, so I'll do my best to keep it within the gap so you don't get a fee. You know, I'll try. At the end of the day, I do need to make a living, but if you get a fee just give me a call and we'll see what we can work out. I'm not here to try and make money off your situation."

I couldn't believe how nice he was being. "Thank you so much. You don't have to do that, but I really appreciate it!" I said happily.

He proceeded to put the cannula into my hand, which was extremely painful. Usually, I'm good with pain, but this was unpleasant to say the least. Poor Tommy hates needles so he couldn't watch, but I'm sure he felt the same pain I did just based on my facial expressions.

It wasn't long before I was being wheeled away. I kissed Tommy goodbye and was wheeled into the operating room. It all happened quickly. The anaesthetist told me what he was doing and that I'd start to feel sleepy as he started the anaesthetic. The next thing I knew I was being wheeled into the recovery room, with Tommy leaning over me saying excitedly, "Hey, bud!"

I was still very woozy and kind of just smiled and closed my eyes. I heard the nurse say, "Give her a few minutes to wake up. I'll go and get some food; she'll need to eat before you can take her home."

Finally, after the drugs started wearing off, I was able to talk. I now understood how Tommy felt every morning when I woke up full of beans and jumped on top of him saying, "Morning, babe!" while he was still half asleep. Waiting for me to come out had been a long 40 or so minutes for Tommy, and he was so happy to see me. Being the patient, you forget that surgery has an impact on other people as well. The nurse came back in with food, and I asked if I could go to the toilet. I felt as though there was a lot of blood and I wanted to put my own pad and underwear on rather than those grotty granny knickers (if you can even call them knickers) they give you for surgery. She obliged and directed me to the toilet.

After a good half an hour in recovery I was sitting up, functioning, and had kept food down, so I was allowed to go home. Tommy walked me out to the car and held my hand the whole way home. Thank God that was now all over. The following day I got a call from Dr A to ask how I was feeling. I had no pain and minimal bleeding, so all in all I was feeling 100 times better than I had felt in the few days leading up to the surgery, and was grateful for the job she'd done. Dr A told me that she'd see me in a week for a post-op consultation, and that she had sent the tissue away for karyotype testing and to check on whether it was a molar pregnancy. She would have the initial findings in a week and the final results would be about six weeks away.

Before my post-op appointment, Mum had told me of a naturopath she had crossed paths with at a conference, who specialised in fertility and recurrent miscarriages. This naturopath had asked Mum if I had been tested for the MTHFR gene, and since I had not, provided a blood referral form for me to go and get a simple blood test to see if I had this gene. Basically, people who have a copy of this gene are unable to metabolise folic acid, which is the synthetic version of folate. Without folate, the risk of miscarriage or birth defects is higher. The results came through, and showed that I had one copy of the MTHFR gene which was C677T. At least now we had some direction on what potentially was causing me to miscarry.

I went to the post-op appointment and took Mum with me. I figured I needed someone to ask medical questions for me. The initial results were fine – it was not a molar pregnancy (from what I researched this was a tumour that could develop as a result of a non-viable pregnancy and had the potential to become cancerous) as previously suspected, and there was no evidence of GTD. Dr A believed it was simply a failed pregnancy that had started to break up, which gave it that "grapey" look. She asked me if I wanted to try to conceive again. I looked at her, looked at Mum, looked back at Dr A, and said, "Yes… if I'm allowed to?"

She laughed and said of course I could. She then proceeded to tell me that until I've had three to four consecutive miscarriages, no real investigation is done. That is bullshit and downright cruel to women. She sympathised with my shock at how many losses I would need to have before further testing would be done, as miscarriage is so common. I distinctly remember her saying, "Some women have nine or more miscarriages, and I honestly don't know how they keep going back." To this day, this statement still pisses me off. We should all be so lucky to not know how or why some women have to keep trying to conceive!

Dr A told me to continue taking folic acid, and I decided to tell her I have a gene that meant I couldn't process it. She knew exactly which gene I was talking about, and found it interesting enough to photocopy the results and add it to my file. What? If you know about this gene, why didn't you suggest I get tested for it? You could have sent me on my merry way for another two or so possible miscarriages before even testing for that? WHAT IS WRONG WITH THE MEDICAL INDUSTRY?

Here is my theory: the reason women need to have multiple miscarriages before investigation is willingly carried out, is because the health system makes too much money from a miscarriage. I'd hate to be right on this, but why else would no one even offer to do some testing until some poor woman has lost multiple babies. That's just sick. Even Dr A herself said that she didn't know how women could keep going back so many times. Then do something about it sooner! It's not rocket science. I wasn't settling for this. I needed answers.

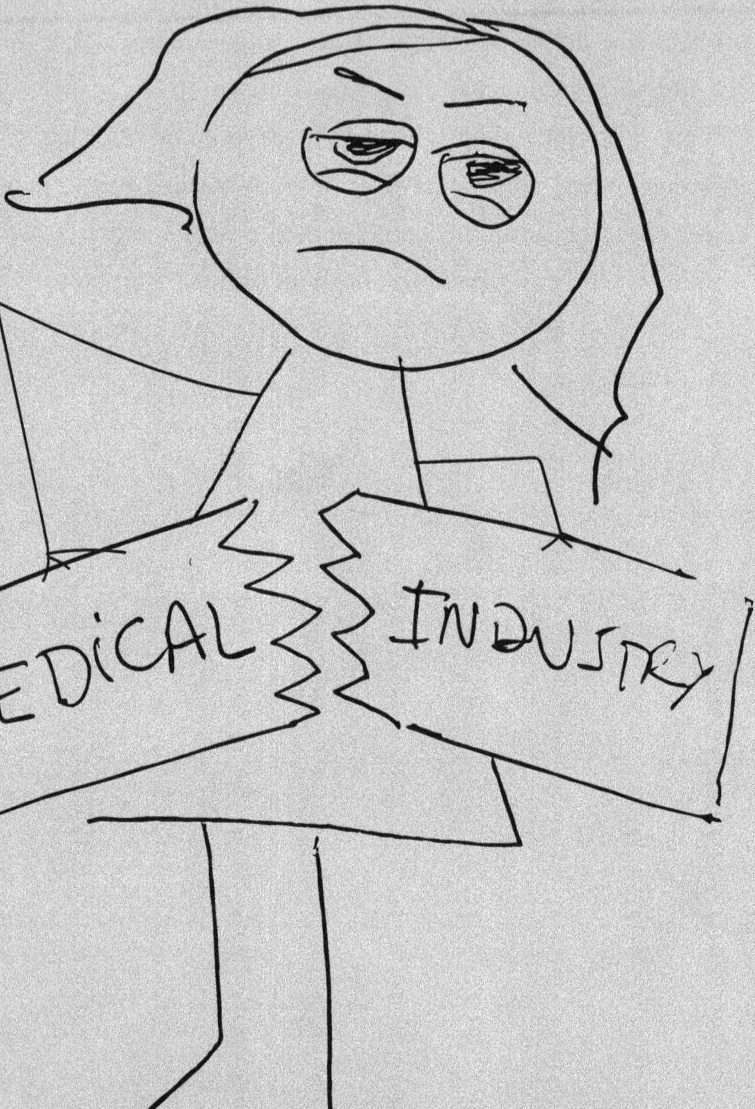
MEDICAL
INDUSTRY

99 VIALS OF BLOOD ON THE WALL

OVER THE NEXT few months, I became very sceptical about the medical industry, and reading a book called *Good Health in the 21st Century* by Dr Carole Hungerford only fuelled that scepticism. I decided to pursue the naturopath my mother had found and had more testing carried out by her, a semen analysis carried out for Tommy, and I also had my GP perform a number of other tests to check possible causes for miscarriage. My GP happened to be a former obstetrician, so she was very thorough in what she tested for.

I think I had about 50 blood tests between May and September 2017. One particular day, I had 10 vials of blood taken. Everything for me came back clear. One test that the naturopath did was for oestrogen, and was to be done on Day 2 or 3 of my period. The results for this showed my oestrogen was quite low, so I was told to drink soy milk to help boost my oestrogen, and to take red clover supplements. I had read another book which explained that sheep in Australia ate red clover and became infertile, and along with that I found a warning on a bottle saying, "Do not consume if you are trying to become pregnant." I gave up on the red clover as I didn't need anything hindering my fertility. Now, I would never have believed that soy milk could make that big a difference to oestrogen levels, until Tommy turned into a bit of an emotional wreck. I made him a coffee every morning, and I used vanilla soy milk in his coffee. Not a great deal, but enough for him to ride the oestrogen dragon – and let's just say he didn't handle it all that well.

Aside from coming out in a rash on his arms, legs and back, he would say things to me like: "I just feel down. All the time. And I don't know why! I have nothing to be sad about. What's wrong with me?" Needless to say, after about a month we stopped drinking soy milk, and he almost immediately felt better and his rash went away. He now warns every man he talks to never to drink soy milk.

The naturopath had us both taking natural supplements which had folate in them, among other things of course. I felt great on these supplements. I felt as though I had more energy and my mental well-being felt better than ever. For as long as I could remember prior to taking the supplements, I had just gotten used to the feeling of never wanting to leave the house or get out of bed, and I'd assumed that's how everyone felt but we all just got on with life. Turns out, because of the gene mutation I have, not getting folate can cause depression and anxiety; I had been medicated for these years earlier but disliked being on medication. Who knew! I was feeling great.

All of the blood tests my GP ordered came back perfect. I didn't have any issues with clotting, and received evidence of perfect health in all other aspects. I got the phone call from Dr A's office to say the karyotype testing came back fine, and Tommy and I were perfectly compatible. This is all great news to most people, but for anyone who has ever had a miscarriage, it's bittersweet. It's great to hear that medically there is nothing wrong. But that doesn't give me answers on why I've had two miscarriages, does it? Tommy's semen analysis came back, and he was happy for the naturopath to give me the results. I skyped with her to discuss it.

"So, there's three main things we look for in semen. Motility, which is the speed of the semen; count, which is the amount of semen per millilitre; and morphology, which is the shape. His count was a little low - he had 10 million per millilitre, and normal count is anything that is more than 20 million. His motility was good; it was 57%, so I'm happy with that. His morphology was only 3%, which means only 3% of his sperm is healthy. The rest have two heads or two tails, or are deformed. So, if one of them fertilises your egg, you will miscarry or have a baby with deformities."

My jaw had dropped and my head was spinning. We needed to stop having sex immediately. Three percent! Not only that, but I was now vividly picturing little swimmers with multiple heads and/or tails. Graphic to say the least.

"In order to fix his morphology, we'll get him taking a high dose herb, which is fairly potent. But it has proven to dramatically improve morphology within three months. We want him to be up at around 30% morphology."

I wrote all the information down and finished my skype session. How on earth was I going to tell Tommy this? While he was still at work, I rang my mother and relayed the news to her. She was in shock as well.

"Maybe you guys are going to seriously need to look into IVF if you want to have children. That way, only the healthy sperm are picked."

I didn't even want to think about this. I hung up the phone and immediately started googling morphology. So did my mother... For most of us, googling is a terrible thing to do. When investigating symptoms or illnesses, in three short clicks we all suddenly have cancer and are sure to die as soon as yesterday. It's a slippery slope. In this case, it was a huge relief. Within minutes my mother and I were texting each other, after finding several different articles stating that the average morphology in semen is 4%. FOUR PERCENT! Why didn't the naturopath lead with this statistic? Sometimes I think people in any form of health profession get some sort of sick enjoyment out of freaking people out. Tommy was 1% less than the average man. And to top that off, one semen analysis isn't even a true indication of what your results are. You need at least three to get true results.

I was now officially put off this naturopath as well. The high-dose potent herb arrived about a week after speaking with her, and Tommy taste tested it. I figured I should probably understand what he was having to take so we both had some. What the naturopath failed to mention was this high-dose herb was BASICALLY PAINT! Oh man, it was so bad. I said then and there that I couldn't make him have this stuff three times a day. I nearly threw it up, and it continued to burn down your throat for hours after having it. No amount of fruit juice, coffee or vodka could get rid of the foul taste in your mouth. You were basically swigging paint and methylated spirits all in one. Just writing this I have my face screwed up and, yep, I actually think I can taste it. Yuck! We were done with the naturopath.

We continued to take our multivitamins twice daily and were having regular sex. I wanted to check when I ovulated again, so I decided to use the sticks in the month of August. It just so happened that this particular month, my body had a bit of a spaz attack and I didn't ovulate until about Day 17 or 18 of my cycle, when previously it had been around Day 13 or 14. By Day 16, I had decided that the surgery had screwed my body up so that I could never ovulate, and I'd never be able to get pregnant. As I said earlier, I do have a tendency to go from zero to one hundred pretty damn quick and I always go to worst-case scenario for myself. It's a gift, I know. In all fairness, Day 16 of this cycle happened to be the anniversary of the twins' due date. They would have been one year old.

Given the date and circumstances and the fragility of my emotions that day, this reaction was kind of warranted. After crying my eyes out, I dusted myself off and decided to just keep doing the ovulation sticks until I ran out in a few days, and then I'd go back to my GP to talk about doing more testing to see why I'd stopped ovulating. The following morning, I got a positive ovulation test. Haha... my bad.

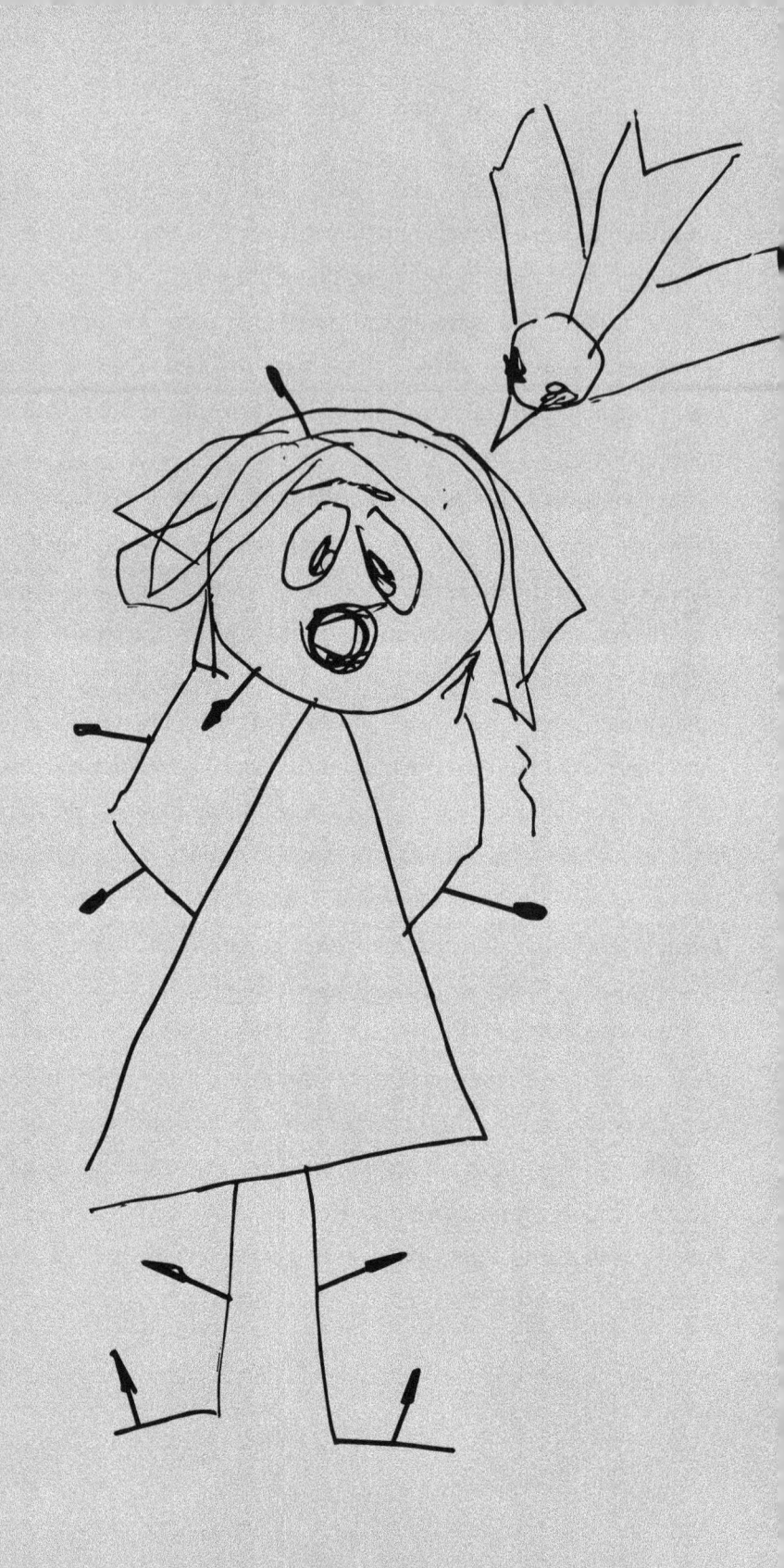

SPECIALISTS AND ACUPUNCTURE

I GOT MY period on September 5th and made the decision to start getting acupuncture. I had heard good things about an acupuncturist who was a local, and figured I had nothing to lose. I also made the decision to be referred to a fertility specialist to see if there was anything else that maybe we could or should be doing, given the fact Tommy had marginally low count and morphology based on the male average. His name was Dr B*.

I got the referral to Dr B and he went through all the bloods I'd had done, the results from my operation, and Tommy's semen analysis. He was a funny old man, very quietly spoken but also very thorough. He disputed my low oestrogen results and told me that on Day 2 or 3 of your period your oestrogen dips quite low, and it peaks during ovulation. This made sense – so of course, it would be low during my period. All that soy milk for nothing! Tommy was less than impressed about that. Dr B ordered another semen analysis for Tommy, and he explained that results for semen can be vastly different based on your health at the time of testing. If you're slightly run down, tired, or not feeling your best, you can get a very poor result. If you're in good health, it can be a great result. Until we had additional data, there was nothing to compare to. He also ordered another karyotype test for us both, just in case we had a third miscarriage and found that to be the cause.

During the initial consultation, he informed us that the baby we lost in May was a female. This was hard to hear. I had never felt like I was pregnant with the last one and the scan showed what looked like an empty sac, so I figured I'd passed it already. But no, what Dr A had extracted and tested was in fact female chromosomes. A baby girl. My heart ached when Dr. B told us ever so casually. I left the appointment and cried. We never knew what gender the twins were, so to now know that we had lost a daughter made the sting and heartache all the more real.

My first acupuncture appointment was great. The acupuncturist was lovely. He ordered a herb for me to start taking three times daily. It didn't taste great, but it was nothing on the paint mixture Tommy had been given, so I was happy to take it. We agreed for me to continue seeing him once a fortnight. Even if I never fell pregnant, just being in his presence was a great feeling. It was all a bit weird. I mean, at one point he basically lit a fire on my belly but hey, I was into it. It made me feel good, so I figured, why not? Tommy, of course, was in full support of whatever made me feel good.

The results from our karyotype testing and Tommy's semen analysis came back, and our compatibility was great. Even better was Tommy's high score with his semen. His count had gone from

10 million to 50 million, and I think from memory his morphology was at 4%. Dr B explained to us that basically 97% of men's semen is rubbish anyway, and only the strongest sperm get through to fertilise the egg. Tommy's count, motility and morphology were fine, so he told us to come back two weeks after a positive home pregnancy test, because there was nothing more fertility-wise he needed to do. We were ecstatic.

It was a few days before my period was due and my boobs had started to get a bit tender. I hadn't had this symptom with my period since the curette in May, so I put it down to the acupuncture and herb starting to sort my body out. Great! I was due to get my period on the 2nd or 3rd of October, and a few months before I had decided that I would only drink when I had my period. I didn't want to risk causing any additional issues if I was lucky enough to fall pregnant again.

Tommy and I had decided to go mountain bike riding this particular Saturday, which was the 30th of September. We hired a bike for me to ride as Tommy already had one. It was quite literally the hottest day of the year thus far. On the way up the mountain, I got bomb dived by a magpie twice, which is a panic-attack-inducing experience for me as I have a debilitating fear of birds. I had a brand-new helmet on and that bastard bird took a chunk out of it. I was hysterical. After Tommy calmed me down, we pushed on up this mountain through 40-degree heat. While riding up this hill, I had a moment of dizziness that made me get off the bike and walk it the rest of the way. At this moment I suddenly thought, "Holy shit, I think I'm pregnant." I didn't say anything to Tommy at the time.

On the way down the mountain, I stupidly found some unwarranted confidence and rode completely outside my ability. I got a little too cocky and slammed the breaks, which resulted in me going over the hangers. I managed to land on my feet somehow, even though one leg got caught between the handlebars and the seat, but it gave me enough of a fright that I decided to walk the bike down the hill, and I made a decision that this mountain biking gig was officially not for me. That night, Tommy and I were sitting outside chatting while he had a beer. I told him that I was going to do a pregnancy test in the morning because it was footy finals the following day, and I wanted to check before I decided to drink. He thought it was a good idea to check before I drank, and that was the last we spoke about it that night.

Now, for anyone who has Snapchat, Tommy and I both have our own animated bitmoji. His is dressed in a Hawaiian t-shirt and there happens to be a bitmoji of a stork delivering a sack, with the bitmoji appearing overly excited for obvious reasons. Tommy sent it to me one day and I asked him if that was how he would react when we finally fell pregnant. He had said to me, "I think I actually will be that excited. I'll be so happy I'll have to put a Hawaiian shirt on and everything!" Well, Sunday the 1st of October I woke up at 5.00am for some stupid reason and was busting to go to the loo. I quickly went into the bathroom to grab a pregnancy test and sleepily aimed for the stick. I left the stick in the bathroom, washed my hands, and went to put the kettle on and let the dog out. After a few minutes, I went back into the bathroom and couldn't believe my eyes when that second line started appearing. I didn't believe it at first and went and sat in front of the TV for a few minutes. It was too good to be true. I went back into the bathroom, expecting there to only be the one negative line and that I'd just imagined that second line was there. But no, there it was. Clear as anything. I was pregnant. We'd done it! Third time lucky. This was it. And it was bloody 5.30 am and Tommy was still asleep. Nooooooooooooooo! I knew he hadn't been sleeping well, so I left him to sleep in. This was no easy feat, let me tell you.

It was after 8.00am when I finally heard him watching videos on his phone. I burst into the bedroom and said to him, "I need you to put a Hawaiian t-shirt on right now."

He looked at me and said, "What?"

I repeated myself and he stared at me as if I was crazy and said, "What the fuck are you on about, Fi?"

I then said, "I need you to put a Hawaiian t-shirt on like your bitmoji, because I'M PREGNANT!"

His eyes lit up and he yelled, "Are you?"

I gave him a big hug and a kiss and ran out to grab the pregnancy test to prove it. "Look!" I said excitedly.

We were both over the moon.

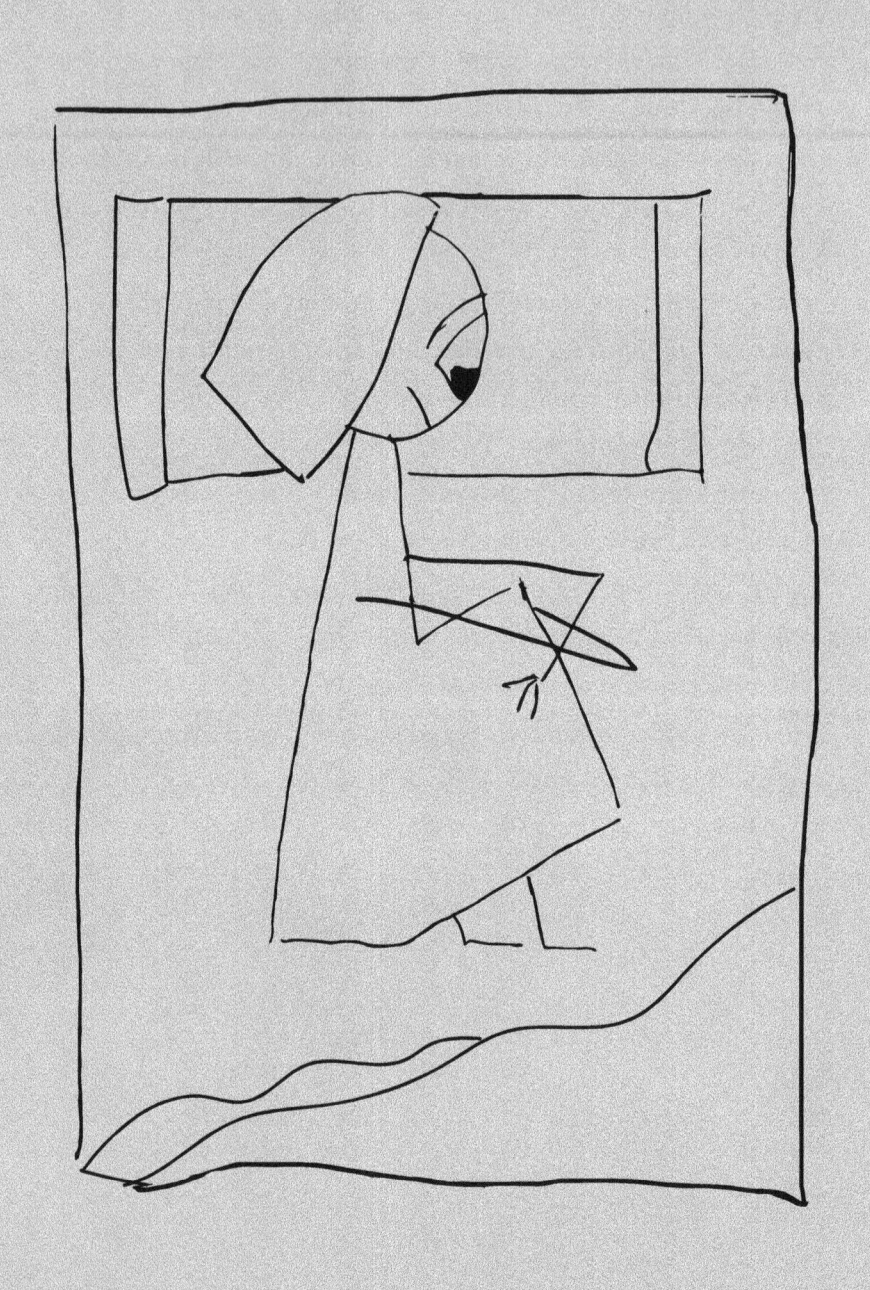

THIRD TIME'S A CHARM

THIS WAS IT. We had done everything right in the lead up to falling pregnant. We were both healthy, had been taking folate for four months, and we'd had all the testing possible to make sure there was nothing wrong with us. We were going to have a baby this time. I contacted Dr B's office and got a script for progesterone. I wanted to make sure I was giving this baby all the help in the world to stick and get nice and comfy in there. I let the acupuncturist know I was pregnant, and he was over the moon for me. Everything was falling into place.

Tommy and I arranged to see Dr B two weeks after I' had the positive pregnancy test, like he'd told us. I was very anxious leading up to this scan. I had worked myself up a few nights beforehand, and convinced myself my boobs weren't even sore anymore and that I'd lost this one too. When I woke up the next morning, Tommy rolled over and grabbed my boob quite hard.

"Ow, dude! What was that for?"

He looked at me and said smartly, "I just wanted to prove a point. They're still sore – you're still pregnant. Stop stressing yourself out."

Well played. In the waiting room to see Dr B, I was so nervous. I had said to Tommy that I felt it was too soon to see a heartbeat and we'd have to wait another week. I'd taken the day off work because I knew I'd be stressed, but I just wanted to get this scan over with.

Dr B called us into the room and performed the scan. On the screen, I could see that everything that should be in my uterus was in there, which calmed me down a lot. It wasn't just an empty sac like last time. Dr B explained that he couldn't see a heartbeat, but we were not to be disheartened as we'd try again next week, and hopefully we'd get one. He said it may just be too early to get a heartbeat. I was calm as we left his office. I felt in my gut that everything was fine, and it was just too soon, and that next week we'd see a heartbeat. I was clinging to hope.

After this appointment I went to my acupuncturist. He was great. He checked my pulse and put my mind at ease. "Your pulse is certainly acting the way a pregnant pulse should. So, I'm thinking it was just too early. You'll get a heartbeat next week, and make sure you let me know how you go." I felt at ease.

The following week, Dr B unfortunately had to cancel our appointment, so my mother's business partner arranged a scan form for us; and we had done more bloods to check on my beta HCG levels. They were steadily rising, which was all a great sign. Tommy met me for the scan, and I was so nervous. I just wanted to see a heartbeat so I could relax. I had to empty my bladder because of course it was too full – and I'd only had 200ml. I looked myself in the mirror in the toilet and said out loud, "You've got this, girlfriend.

You're about to see a heartbeat. Just relax." I was trying to give myself a pep talk before going back in.

I got back in the room and the woman doing my scan turned the machine so I could see the screen. She inserted the probe into my vagina and up appeared my uterus. Before she could even say anything, I saw that beautiful flickering heart and said, "Oh my god, there it is!" I had tears rolling down my face I was so happy to see that amazing heart pumping away so strongly.

"Where is it?" Tommy asked desperately.

The woman zoomed in closer and pointed to the screen showing our baby's heart pumping away at 111 beats per minute. Amazing. The baby was measuring at six weeks and two days, giving us a due date of June 19th 2018. I was completely over the moon.

We got out of the scan and texted a picture to my mother and she rang us, so happy that we'd gotten a heartbeat. Hooray! This was it. Tommy and I went to grab a bite to eat in celebration and while we waited for our food I was dancing around, so happy. We'd done it. I can remember texting my mother later saying, "Go me and my uterus!" and I meant it. I was so damn proud of the fact that I had a healthy baby growing in my belly after going through two very traumatic miscarriages.

On Thursday November 2nd I had my normal fortnightly appointment with my acupuncturist. He was thrilled that I'd let him know we'd had a heartbeat, and we carried on with acupuncture. I remember lying there while he checked my pulse, and he made a face that resembled confusion. I didn't say anything at the time, but wondered if he could tell something that I couldn't. We carried on with the appointment and as I left, he said to me, "Okay, well I'll see you in a fortnight. And just remember – positive thoughts." He gestured to his stomach to encourage me to send positive vibes to the baby. Looking back on it, I think he could tell from my pulse that something was wrong.

The following evening after Tommy and I had sex, I went to the toilet and saw bright red blood. "

Oh no. No no no no no no! It's okay. Calm down. It's not a lot. Everything will be okay." I was talking to myself in the toilet.

I came out and said to Tommy, "Okay, so I've just had a bit of a bleed. I've put a pad on just in case. It wasn't a lot; I was just shocked to see it. I'm not in pain or anything…"

Tommy remained calm and told me that it can happen after sex and that there's probably nothing wrong. He'd obviously done plenty of his own research in the past, and his calm attitude kept me calm. I messaged my mother and she reassured me that with no pain it's usually a good sign. She told me to keep an eye on it, and if I had no more bleeding maybe the progesterone had caused a build-up of blood vessels in my vagina and sex had just irritated them. I was officially put off sex until after our next scan. Sorry, Tommy!

I made it through the weekend constantly feeling my boobs, which still felt tender. I was still hungry so I tried my hardest to relax. By Monday night I was a complete mess. It felt like my boobs had started to shrink, but I'd had no more bleeding and certainly no pain. I hardly slept on the Monday night and woke up on Tuesday morning to see I had lost 0.2g on the scales. Well, this tipped me over the edge. I needed a scan and I needed it today. I just needed to see that everything was fine. I felt as though it was, but I couldn't wait another four weeks for the 12-week scan – I'd send myself crazy! Mum was again out of town, which she always seemed to be when these things happen; but she told me to ring for an emergency appointment with my GP and to call the sonographer and book the appointment for the same day. I went to see my GP at 8.30am, and she was more than happy to give me blood test forms and a scan referral. She told me to relax as much as I could, and said we would know soon enough.

I went and did my bloods, and my scan was scheduled for 12:45pm. I picked Tommy up for the scan so he could be with me. I was so glad he had come to every single aspect of this pregnancy; he was such a great support. Sitting in the waiting room, I was calm. I had no indication that anything was wrong and felt as though I had just worked myself up, which given my history was completely understandable. My name was called and the girl doing my scan was the same lady who had completed my scan at the hospital with my last miscarriage. I was glad it was her. We got into a small, pokey room which had a small screen monitor and a short probe line.

She said to me, "I'm just going to bring everything up on the screen and have a look, then I'll talk you through it." Because I felt like it was all going to be okay, I was fine with that. How wrong I was.

Within seconds of my uterus coming into view, the girl asked me, "Did they get a heartbeat when you came two weeks ago?" I told her yes, and confirmed the due date of 19th June based on the previous scan. Her next words cut like a knife. "Okay. Fiona, I'm not getting a heartbeat and the baby is still measuring six weeks two days, so there's been no growth since your last scan. I'm so sorry. I'll just take a couple of pictures and then I'll let you get changed. When are you seeing your doctor?"

I stared at her and went into autopilot. "Okay, no worries. I'll see her tomorrow morning."

I stared at the ceiling while she finished taking photos of my uterus and lifeless baby. I couldn't believe it. I was in shock. How had this happened a third time? This was supposed to be the one. Our rainbow baby. Our miracle. Why was it gone? There was nothing medically wrong with us, so it just didn't make sense. I started to get angry.

The girl left the room. She'd told me I could leave straight away and didn't need to see the staff at the front desk. Thank God. After she walked out of the room, I looked at Tommy. He was in shock.

"I'm so sorry, babe. I didn't expect that at all," he said, looking pale and confused.

"Neither did I," I said. And I really didn't.

We walked out of the room and got in the car. I texted my mother: "No heartbeat and still measuring 6w 2 days. Don't ring. Not ready to talk."

We drove home in complete silence. Tommy held my hand and lovingly rubbed it. There was nothing to say. This was fucked. I dropped Tommy off at his truck so he could drive it home, and it gave me a minute to get home before him and scream into a pillow. I wanted to break things.

All the same questions came flooding back. How had this happened a third fucking time? Were we just not meant to have kids, and this was the world's way of telling us to give it up? Was I really going to be that shit of a mother that my uterus felt the need to kill my baby every time I tried to bring one into the world? Why had we bothered jumping through all these hoops, just for our pregnancy to fail again? I was pissed the fuck off and I needed a drink. I poured myself a large glass of wine and enjoyed every damn drop of it.

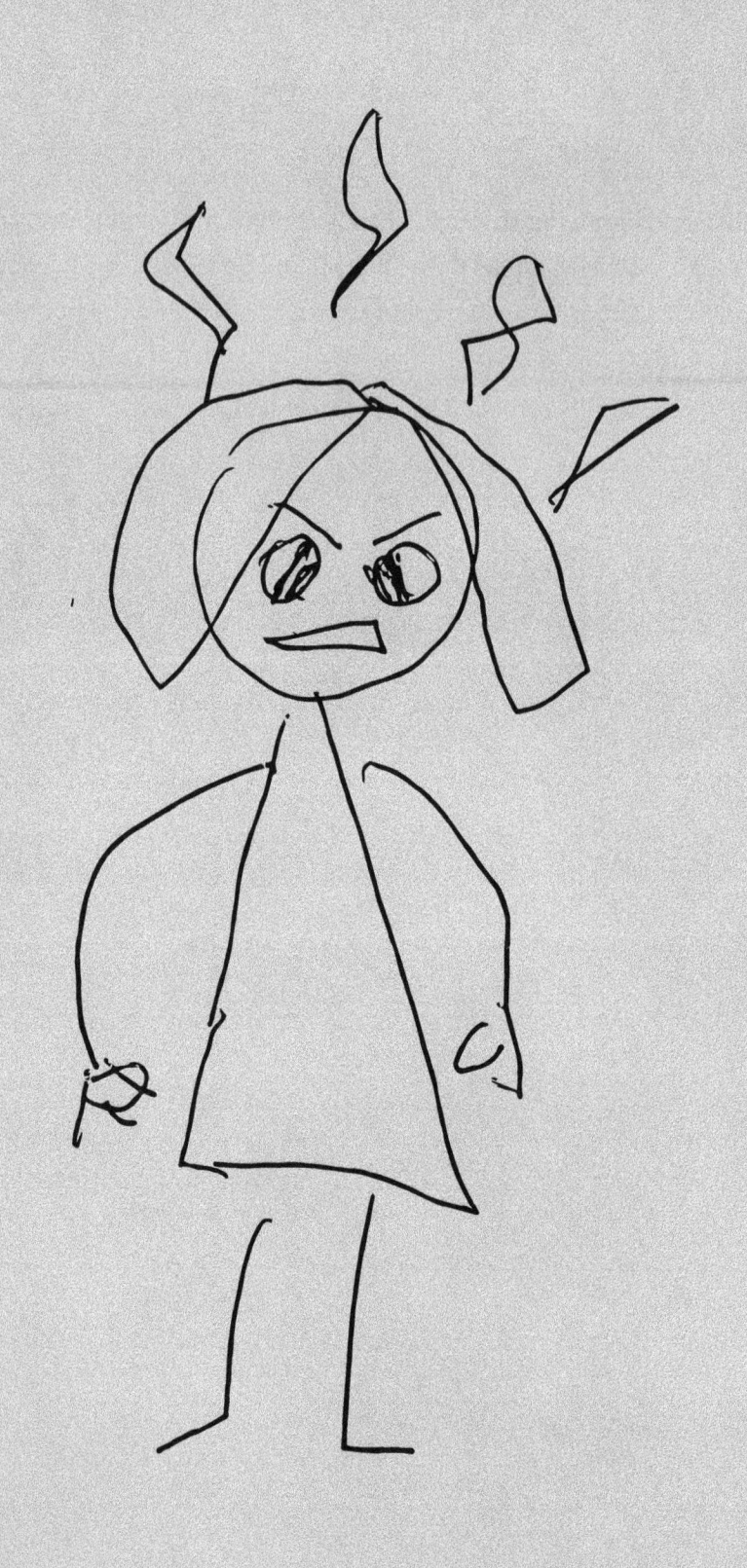

DING, DING, DING; ROUND THREE

I'D BOOKED AN appointment to see my doctor at 10:45am the following morning. I had what I was going to say. I wanted to get all the information out before she could say anything to me, because I just couldn't deal with how lovely she would be. Tommy took the remainder of the week off to be with me, which looking back, we both needed more than we realised. He came into the appointment with me, and we both sat down.

"So, the scan yesterday didn't go well. There was no heartbeat, and the baby was still measuring the same as the first scan at 6 weeks 2 days, so its heart must have stopped the same day as the last scan. I'm hoping you can refer me to Dr A again, and I'll call today once the referral has been sent through so I can get this happening as fast as possible." Success. I got it all out, no tears, and absolutely nailed the delivery. Go me.

My doctor looked at me, gave an uncomfortable laugh and decided to talk directly to Tommy. "You know, Fiona is an amazing woman. So courageous. I am the doctor, and I do not like delivering results such as these, but she has come in here and made my job so easy by telling me the results, which is what I should be doing. So thank you, Fiona, for making my job easier. You're just so brave."

Oh dear. Tommy laughed and rubbed my back. Here come the tears. Why does she have to say such lovely things? I had nailed my speech and now I'd turned into the pathetic sloppy mess that I didn't want to be. Dammit!

"Okay, so you have both discussed that you want to have medical intervention?" she asked politely. We had. We just wanted to get this over with so we could get on with our lives.

I got the referral sent through to Dr A, then my doctor told me that this was her second last week here as she would be moving towns the following week. What? No! I think I was more upset that I was losing her as my GP than I was that I'd had a third miscarriage.

She said to me gently, "Fiona, I know right now it doesn't seem like it, but you will go on to have a successful pregnancy. And I will be waiting to hear the good news. I want you to have my phone number, and please call me any time you want to ask questions or need advice about this sort of thing in the future." She hugged me as I left. Man, this was heartbreaking.

I called Dr A's office to be told that she was out of town, and I would need to get my referral sent to Dr C*, who was looking after Dr A's patients while she was away. I got the referral changed and contacted Dr C's office. My appointment was scheduled for 3.30pm on Thursday 9th November with Dr C, and I was to fast from 11:00am just in case he decided to perform the surgery that evening after he finished his practice for the day. Awesome. Tommy and I went to have lunch at a pub and we both ordered ourselves a well-deserved beer. The beer went down way too well so we thought stuff it, we'll grab a carton of beer on the way home and just get pissed. When we got home, we managed to convince Tommy's mum to give up what she was doing and join us for an afternoon of drinking. She was easily persuaded, and we cracked open the drinks.

That was a great afternoon. We managed to dust off two cartons of beer between the three of us and when Tommy's dad got home from work, he joined us too. His parents were so sad for us, but they understood not to hug me or be sad for us because everyone else's pain was just too much for me to deal with. I'm pretty good at handling my own shit, but seeing how hurt everyone else is breaks my heart and breaks me down. Just keep your pain to yourself because I'm already in enough of my own!

The hardest part of losing this baby was watching the way it rolled Tommy. He had been part of every single aspect of this baby, and losing it rocked him to the core. He was so excited for this baby and more than ready to be an amazing father, only to have it taken away from him so abruptly. I was glad that he had the week off; it gave him the chance to talk things through and not have to get straight back into work. He needed the break. Three miscarriages, two in less than six months, had taken their toll on Tommy. I could see it in his eyes.

Thursday rolled around and I wasn't hungover. Winning! I took the dog for a walk and ate as much food as I could until about 11.00am, from which time I had to fast. We made it to our appointment and met Dr C for the first time. He was lovely; my kind of doctor – black and white with information. He went through my referral from my GP and proceeded to tell me what we test for once women have had three miscarriages.

"I've already been tested for everything," I said. "We've had karyotype testing performed twice, I have no issues with clotting, and all other tests came back fine."

He looked at me. "Oh! Well then, you're just…"

"Unlucky?" I finished his sentence.

He nodded. He proceeded to tell us there was nothing medically wrong with either of us and there was nothing more that needed to be tested. We knew all this. We were now officially in the "unexplained" category which, to be honest, is an ordinary place to be. On the one hand it's amazing that there's nothing wrong with us, but on the other hand it's not a fucking answer or outcome. It's nothing. It's limbo.

We headed over to the hospital and were told to come back at about 5.00pm to be admitted. We ducked around to my mum's house to fill in time, and we were distracted by my niece and nephew being there which was great. Shortly before 5.00pm, we returned to the hospital to check in. I was led to the maternity ward, which was the last place I wanted to be. Having just had my third miscarriage, I didn't want to be anywhere near babies or other people who were happy with their healthy bundles of joy. I sucked it up and got into my bed. The nurse looking after me was a dithery old bat, but she really was quite lovely. She gave me my gown and feral surgery knickers and told me to have a shower with special soap. I had been told that they were running late in theatre, and I was the second one to be done so shouldn't expect to go in until at least 8.30/9.00pm. Great. I wasn't starving or anything.

I encouraged Tommy to head off and get himself some food while I showered and got myself ready. I had just begun to bleed as I got in the shower. I was so angry that I was in this position again. It was bullshit. I got a bit teary in the shower because I was so exhausted by this whole process. Conception, scans, folate, progesterone, acupuncture, specialists, the works. All for nothing. I was done. I didn't want to think about babies or pregnancy for a very long time. Tommy still wasn't back from getting food when a gentleman came into the room and said he was taking me down to surgery. What? No! I hadn't said goodbye to Tommy. I quickly texted him to say that they were taking me down and that I loved him. As they wheeled me out, he came skidding into the room to say goodbye to me. Phew! I'm glad he made it.

The operating room this time was a lot more overwhelming than last time. I had people barking orders at me to give my full name, date of birth, explain what procedure I was having done, and who was performing the operation. Meanwhile, I had an anaesthetist telling me he was putting a cannula in and a theatre nurse telling me she was sticking monitors to my head and that they would hurt when she pushed them to stick to my skin. Back to the anaesthetist telling me what he was putting into me. Back to a nurse telling me she was putting more monitors on my chest. I could feel myself becoming woozy. Hurry up, let me pass out. I don't want to be here.

I woke up still in the theatre area with the nurse talking to me. I asked her if I could lie on my side. I was in excruciating pain. "Uhhh. I suppose that would be okay." She ran it by someone else, but I didn't care, I was lying on my side. They kept me down near theatre until I was much more awake, and then wheeled me back up to maternity ward.

I tried to appear excited to see Tommy, which in all fairness I was. The poor guy had chewed his nails down so much that a few of them were bleeding. He was so happy I was out. After about 40 minutes and a piece of raisin toast, I was allowed to go home. Tommy had to hold me while we were walking out because I felt very wobbly. He had ordered me KFC while I was in surgery, and had left it at Mum's house to be reheated for me to eat on the drive home. Legends! I inhaled the KFC on the drive home and was so happy to crawl into bed. Normally, we're not cuddlers, but that night I fell asleep completely cuddled into Tommy and I've never felt more at home. As weird as it sounds, everything just felt right in the world. It was all over, and we could get on the road to recovery.

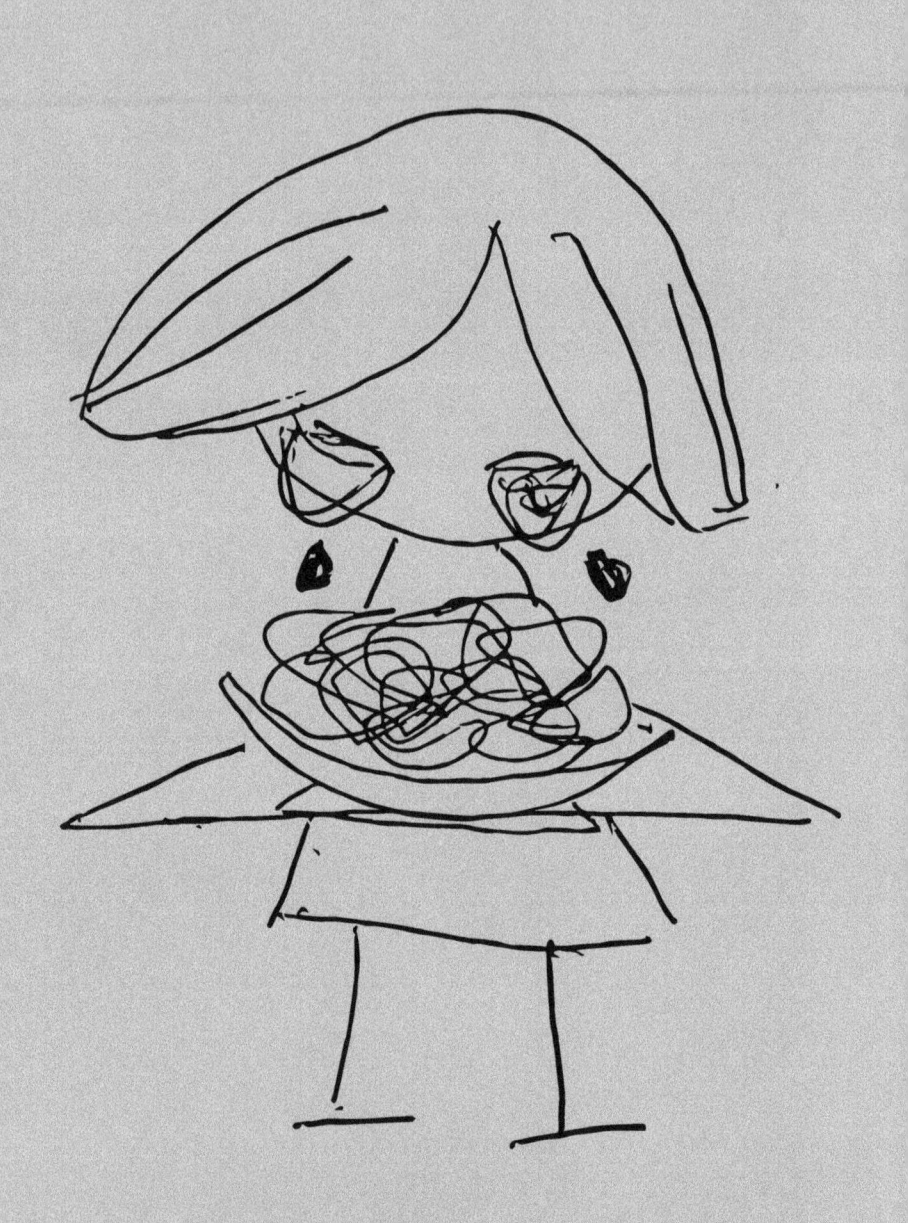

POST-OP FUN

FRIDAY. THE DAY after surgery. I felt amazing. Tommy, on the other hand, was one flat human and I just couldn't get him out of his unhappy black hole. This continued into Saturday. The poor guy just wasn't in a good place. He was over-sleeping and then he just felt down all day. It was understandable, but no one ever thinks about how much the man suffers as well. I was certainly guilty of forgetting to make sure he's okay through all these miscarriages. But I'd made a conscious effort to be there for him with this one, because out of the two of us, I was handling it better. I think I'd just become numb.

Tommy got back into his mountain bike riding and managed to feel a bit better by Saturday lunchtime. We decided to go and meet up with one of his mates who was having a day by a local lake. We took some beers and headed off. When we got there, his mate had the biggest smile on his face, and his girlfriend came running over to me saying, "The best thing ever just happened to me!" She was holding up a huge engagement ring. I screamed and hugged her and ran to hug him. It was so exciting. Tommy and I will forever be grateful for being included in their engagement. It had literally happened seconds before, so I'm glad we didn't interrupt. But it was also a great opportunity to get our minds off feeling sorry for ourselves and revel in someone else's happiness.

After spending a few hours with these friends, we opted to go to another friend's house for some more drinks. Tommy had stopped drinking and let me continue on the beers. He wanted to be able to talk to his mate and go through everything with him. So we left them to it while my girlfriend and I managed to get quite silly. It was bloody great.

I woke up on Sunday morning without a hangover, which I was happy about. But I did feel quite flat. By mid-morning I had a fair amount of period pain, but I was trying to ignore it. An additional issue I had with this curette was a very metallic smell coming from my vagina. I don't know how else to explain it, but it almost smelt like burnt flesh. I only noticed it when I sat down to go to the toilet; very bizarre. Tommy had to go down the paddock and help his dad with a piece of machinery. So I decided to start cooking his lunches for the week, because I certainly wasn't going to work. I was trying a new recipe that Tommy had sent me which was lasagne-stuffed noodles. It was stuffed with mushroom, spinach, ricotta, cheese and other good things. Now, I just assumed that you cook lasagne sheets like you would cook pasta. Not so much! After stuffing up the first packet of nine sheets, I decided to try the second packet and cook each sheet of lasagne individually. Even this didn't help.

Out of 18 sheets of lasagne, I successfully cooked five that didn't split and rip and turn to absolute shit. I was devastated. When Tommy arrived back, he taste-tested the stuffing mix. He isn't a fan of mushrooms to begin with, but cold cooked mushrooms nearly made him throw up, and getting them down made him gag. This didn't help me. I stormed off to the bedroom and just lay there crying. He came in to ask what was wrong and apologised for his reaction. He said that he didn't like mushrooms on their own but was sure the food would taste nice.

I started crying quite hysterically and said, "I'm not crying because of you. I'm crying because I fucked up the pasta. And who cries over fucking pasta!"

He started laughing and pulled me in for a big hug. "Just remember you've got a lot of hormones going on, babe, and this is completely normal."

I continued crying into his chest over pasta. Ahhhhh, the post-operation hormonal imbalance fun.

I wanted to try cooking another recipe that needed fresh dill. I said to Tommy that I had forgotten to buy it, so I would have to wait until tomorrow to cook it. He looked at me with one raised eyebrow and said, "Are you sure we don't have dill, Fiona?"

I angrily said no, that I'd already looked for it and we definitely didn't have any.

He had a devilish smile on his face and said, "Okay. I'm just going to have a quick look for it. And if I find the dill, we're renaming it Fiona..."

How mean is that? I mean, it made me giggle, and to be honest I needed that kind of humour in my life; but man, talk about timing. He came strutting back into the room proud as punch, laughing and holding up fresh dill.

I burst into tears again and said, "We're not renaming it!"

He just laughed at me and scooped me up into a hug. I regathered myself, and obviously for quite some time we made jokes over the fact that I'd lost my marbles over bloody pasta, and the dill was now officially called Fiona. But it was a pretty good indication that I wasn't ready to go back to work and that I still needed time to recover from the operation and let my body get back to normal.

About a week after the operation, I had my follow-up appointment with Dr C; by this time the metallic smell had disappeared so I never thought to mention it. I hadn't recalled if I had asked Dr C prior to surgery if the removed product was to be sent away for testing. Once we were in his office, he asked how my recovery was going and if I'd had much bleeding or pain since the procedure, to which I was happy to answer no. He advised that he had not sent the product away for testing and reminded me of our conversation that no further testing needed to be carried out, as there was nothing medically wrong with us.

"Unfortunately, you are just another statistic." I remember these words clearly. Dr C was very positive that I would go on to have a successful pregnancy and recommended I see him as a patient once I was pregnant.

I can remember leaving his office feeling a sense of clarity. There was nothing wrong with Tommy or me, so this was just something we had to accept as part of our journey. We were just another statistic, along with many couples who suffer from recurrent miscarriage.

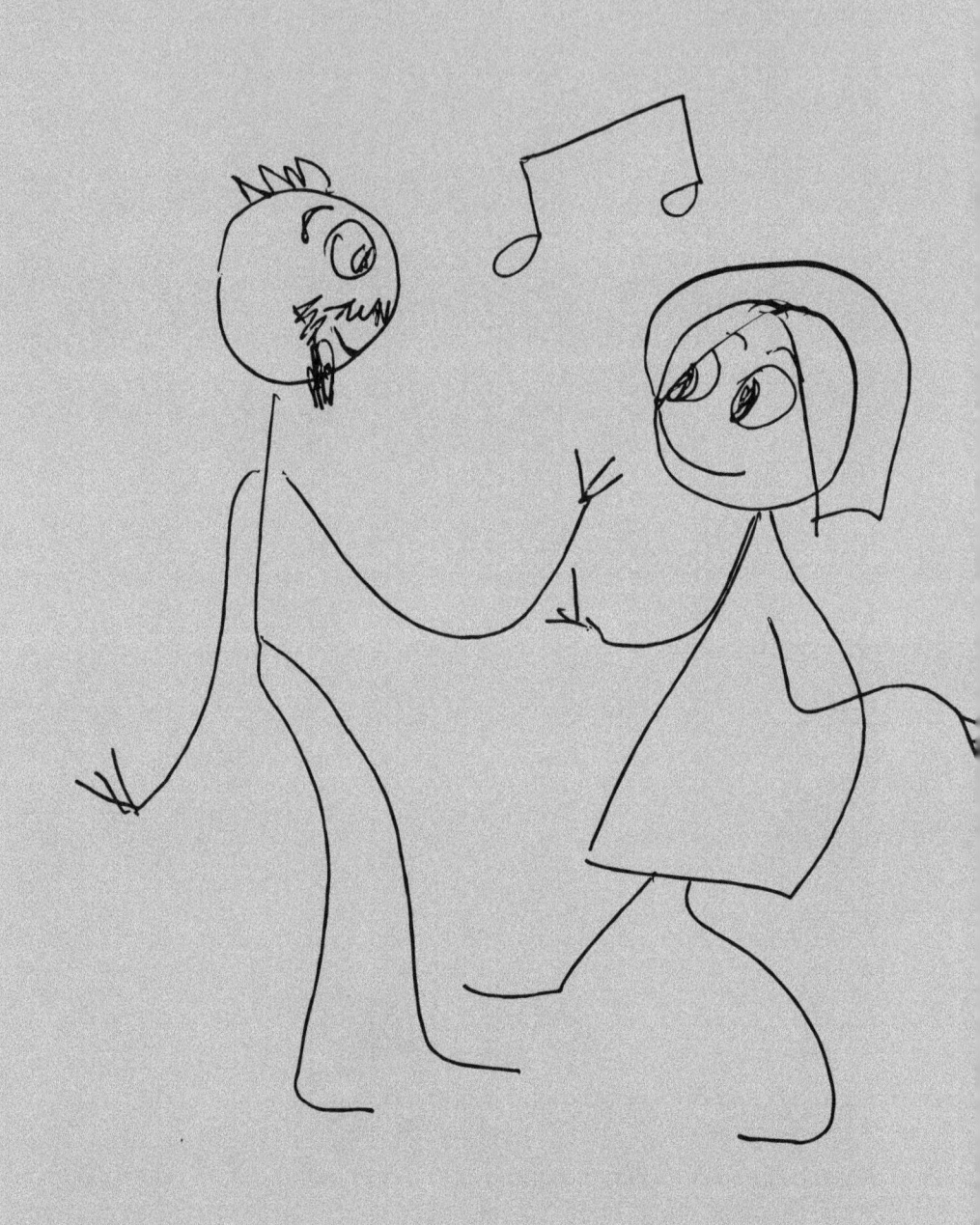

PART 2
THE YEAR OF YES

BY THIS TIME, it was December 2017. We had so much to look forward to. It was almost Christmas, which happens to be my absolute favourite time of the year, and this year we were spending it with my family. We all travelled to a caravan park, where we all spent almost a week in our caravans. Days were spent drinking, eating, and swimming. Tommy and I had decided we were done with trying to have kids. We were looking forward to 2018 and made a pact that it would be The Year of Yes. We would say yes to going on more holidays, doing more fun things, focusing on being completely and utterly selfish by doing exactly what we wanted. We were excited for it.

After my previous miscarriages, my cycle had returned relatively normally. I would say I had more period pain, but I could never 100% say for sure that I was actually in more pain, or if it was a bit of emotional pain more than physical. Looking back, it was definitely physical. Apart from being a hypochondriac, on the other end of the scale I also have a habit of convincing myself that pain is all in my head and there is nothing actually wrong with me. Something I'm trying to work on.

About four weeks after the surgery for my miscarriage in November, period pain reared its ugly head. Great. This meant I would be able to start tracking my cycle to ensure we didn't have sex during my fertile time, as both of us were completely uninterested in going down that path again. Something strange happened, though. I was suffering from severe period pain but getting no bleeding. Bizarre. I didn't think much of it at the time. I remember mentioning it to my mother, who looked a bit confused by it; but we both put it down to my body going through a lot of trauma in the past 18 months and guessed it was a one-off.

In January 2018, I was lucky enough to be given a fantastic opportunity through work to travel to a secluded island and live there for two weeks, carrying out work in the community. Whilst working in this remote community for two weeks, I again suffered extreme period pain for two or three days. I can remember having lunch on a particular day and I couldn't even eat, I was in so much pain. Surely I was going to bleed with this much pain? But no, once again, bang on 29 days after my last bout of pain and no bleeding, I was getting a "period" with no bleeding. What was happening?

Upon my return home, I decided to do some research as to what could possibly be going on. I returned to seeing my acupuncturist, who prescribed me a herb which was to help my period return. I remember thinking that I was getting the pain, but nothing was coming out, so it must be blocked. I had found online a rare condition called Asherman's Syndrome, which matched perfectly with my symptoms and previous history of multiple uterine traumas as well as having an infection in my teens (which I noted in Part 1). I mentioned this condition to my mother who kind of stared at me blankly, having never heard of it. She encouraged me to see a doctor about my period pain and lack of bleeding, though.

Unfortunately, my GP had relocated so my mother recommended another lovely GP who also had practiced as an obstetrician at the hospital. I booked an appointment with her to see what might be happening. I asked Mum to come with me to the appointment. For some reason, seeing someone new felt quite stressful given I had been through so much with my previous GP; I was extremely nervous about building a new relationship with a new doctor. I had all my test results and history in a blue folder under my arm, and waited for my name to be called.

Dr D* was a small woman in a brightly coloured dress. She called my name, spotted my mother when she stood up with me, and lit up when she realised I was her daughter. I handed my folder over to Dr D and explained my history in brief.

After getting through my current symptoms, I said, "I know you probably hate hearing your patients say they have been on google. But I'm wondering if it is possible that I have Asherman's Syndrome? In no way do I think it has been caused by the doctors performing my D&Cs (dilation and curette). My symptoms just seem to match it to a tee!"

She looked at me, then looked at Mum and said matter-of-factly, "No. It's not possible. Asherman's is such a rare condition and it is more likely to occur in women who have had nine or ten procedures done by less experienced doctors. Those who have performed your D&Cs have a wealth of experience, and would not have caused this type of damage. I would suggest you wait a few more weeks and see if you get your period. If not, come back and see me. In the meantime, I will book you for a scan just in case there is some sort of blockage."

Okay. I was happy that she was at least willing to investigate by way of a scan to see if anything was going on, because what I had been experiencing was not normal and I knew it. I was happy with my new GP. She felt a lot more matter-of-fact about what I had been through which, as I've said, I need. I honestly hate it when doctors or nurses soften their voices or get all empathetic on me. No. Get a backbone and just deliver this blow as if you're talking to a brick wall. I do realise that not everyone is like this and health professionals do an exceptional job at dealing with all different types of people; but for me, I can't handle it when news is delivered gently. I knew she was going to be a perfect fit for me.

I continued to receive acupuncture and take the herb that seemed to be doing nothing in bringing a period on. I attended an internal scan, which showed everything looking great. As much as I was happy that everything looked good, it still didn't explain what the hell was going on. This seemed to be the story of my life. After having a third round of extreme period pain, so bad in fact that I remember taking a day off work, I was over it. Back to Dr D to sort it out. I showed up in her office to get the results of my scan, which she was happy with.

"Is there some sort of medication I can take to bring my period on? I've had more period pain and no bleeding, and I just want my period back."

By this point, I was wanting to travel to another State to see a specialist in Natural Killer (NK) cell testing. This had to be done on a certain day in your cycle and because I wasn't technically having a cycle, I couldn't book in with them. Frustrating to say the least.

"No problem. Take this medication. One tablet twice daily for five days and then you will get your period a few days later." Dr D gave me a script and sent me on my merry way.

I took those tablets religiously. I have never wanted to get my period so badly in all my life! Finally, on 14th February 2018. I got my first period in almost four months. Whilst it was extremely painful, I was thrilled. As I mentioned, I had been in contact with an NK cell testing clinic and had a temporary appointment for April. I did not want to risk getting pregnant before then, because in my head I was just going to miscarry again, and I was done with that. I purchased some ovulation sticks and tracked my cycle religiously to ensure that we did not have sex during my fertile window, as well as to track what day in my cycle I ovulated.

I received a positive ovulation test on a Thursday morning, and that night we were heading away camping for the weekend with our friends. Tommy and I both made sure we did not have sex for the next two days, just to be sure. The weekend we had away was quite honestly one of the best weekends we had had in a while. Our van was right beside our friends, and they had their two little girls with them, whom we adored. There was a lot of alcohol consumed that weekend and so many laughs, that I think we needed more than ever. It felt like we were back to our old selves.

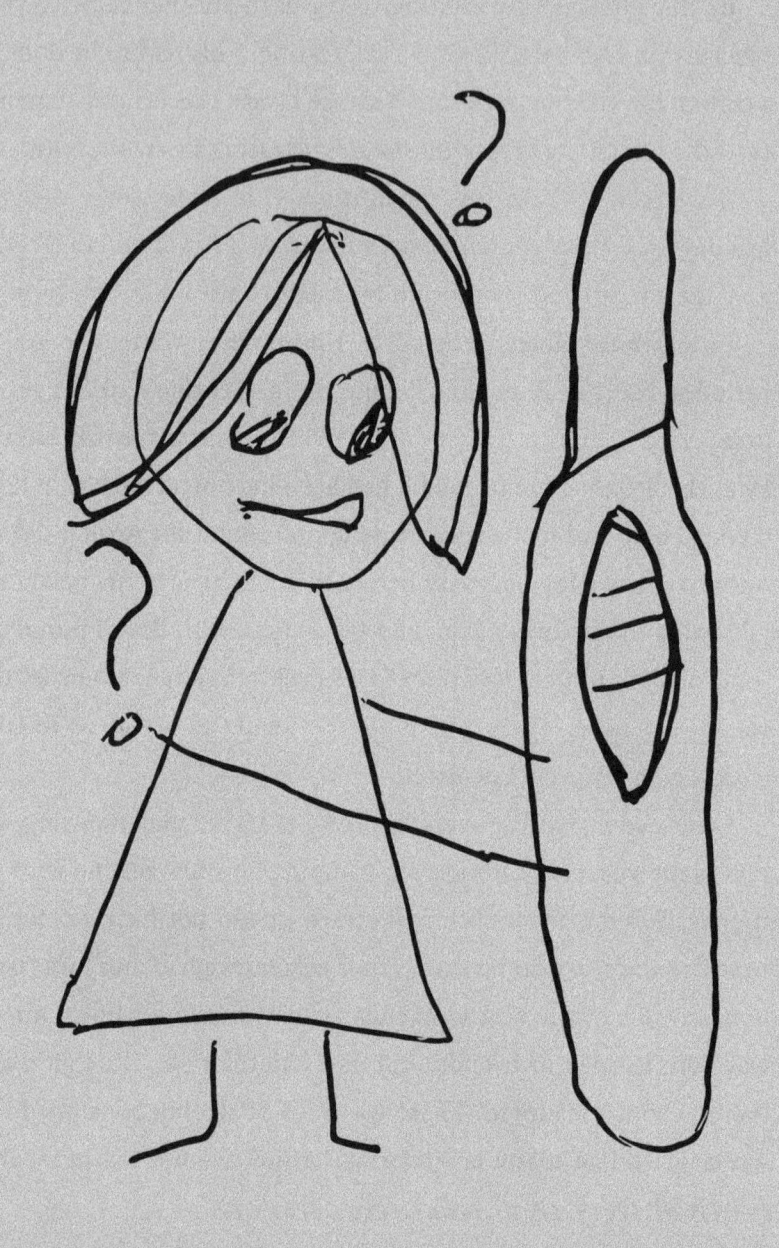

WELL, THAT WAS UNEXPECTED

ON TUESDAY 13TH March, I had no pain but there was bright red blood when I wiped after going to the toilet. Spot on! 28 days after my period, I was bleeding again. Unreal. I put a tampon in and carried on with my business for the day. I remember thinking it was strange that I had no period pain; but I didn't really care because I had blood – the one thing I had been lacking previously – so to me all was well. Interestingly, when I went to change my tampon later that day it came out completely clean. Weird. Oh well, I'd had a bleed, so maybe this was my new normal with periods. I didn't bother wearing a panty liner because I figured it was over.

That Thursday, we travelled with three of our mates to CMC 2018. It was the first time we had been, and we were lucky that our mates had other friends who had pulled out. Since it was The Year of Yes, we jumped on the opportunity. CMC was hands down one of the best festivals of my life. Somehow our van was the party van.

People camped behind us brought their beer bong over, and Tommy invented a "kick the flap" drinking game. Honestly, it's too much to explain, but basically it involves drunk idiots trying to kick the flap of the awning on the caravan. Hilarious!

After four nights and three days of solid drinking, it was time to go home. We were all a bit worse for wear on the Monday, and being the worst map reader in history, I sent us on a wild goose chase which added an extra few hours to our drive home. With everyone so hungover, I was really popular, as you can imagine. While we were driving home, Mum sent me a text asking if I'd got my period. I replied saying I had a super light bleed the week before, but it only lasted a few hours and it was all over with.

Her response made me feel sick. "You don't think it could be an implantation bleed, do you?"

I replied with, "I don't even want to think about that! I'll do a test when I get home to be sure, but I have no symptoms so I'm sure its fine."

And I didn't. With my previous three pregnancies, my first indication was that I had extremely sore breasts and was visiting the toilet non-stop to wee. Plus, we had been actively trying not to get pregnant, so it just wasn't possible.

When we got home, I did a pregnancy test just to be sure. By the time I had set the pregnancy test down, wiped, pulled my underwear up and flushed the toilet, it was the most positive pregnancy test I had ever seen. And trust me, I'd seen a few. I stormed out of the toilet and angrily thrust the positive test into Tommy's face.

"What the actual fuck!"

He looked at the test and looked at me, a little unsure how to react. "Well, that's exciting?"

"No, it friggen isn't. I'm just going to lose it again."

I was furious. We had done everything to ensure we did not have sex around ovulation, I had a temporary appointment in another State for further testing, and now I was back at square one – basically, waiting for a miscarriage to happen. Awesome. I was pissed the hell off that I'd had a positive test. I chose not to text my mother and put myself to bed in a huff.

The following afternoon, I had an appointment with my acupuncturist. He asked me if I'd got my period again after having it return the month before. "

No," I said rather rudely. "I got a positive pregnancy test, though."

He looked at me and felt my pulse. "You sure did! That's a good pulse."

We continued with the session. I could feel myself detaching from my body, not wanting to be happy about being pregnant because I got burnt every time. I was going to lose it, so best not to get excited about it.

After my appointment, I was heading around to my sister's house to visit and discuss our upcoming family trip for the Easter holidays. My mother happened to be there and I was trying to avoid her because I knew what she wanted to know.

After a little while, she cornered me and discreetly asked, "So did your acupuncturist have any insights on why you only had such a light bleed last week?"

I stared at her and said, "Yep. I'm pregnant." Her jaw dropped.

"What's happened?" My older sister came bustling in asking what was wrong.

I looked at her and said abruptly, "Well, you're going to find out next week when we go away, anyway. I'm pregnant."

Her response matched how I was feeling. "Oh get fucked, dude!" Yep. I agreed.

To this day, my sister still feels awful for her response, but at the time it was exactly how I was feeling about the situation; and my entire family had seen me absolutely broken after all my miscarriages, so for them, it was a struggle of a journey as well.

"Are you okay?" she asked me.

"No, I'm not. I'm pissed off about it. We did everything to not be pregnant and I'm still fucking pregnant; it's bullshit!"

Now, I do regret how angry I was. And I also regret feeling this way about falling pregnant so easily. I know first-hand what it feels like to try your hardest to fall pregnant every single cycle only to get your period. So taking it for granted like this and being so furious about it is not one of my proudest moments. However, given what I had been through, I feel as though it was warranted at the time.

"I'm just not even going to think about it. Let's go on this holiday and I'll deal with it when I come back." And so, we did.

The holiday came at the right time. We headed off in our caravans with my two sisters and their families, and our friends with their two little girls. It was awesome. I started to experience morning sickness, which I hadn't had with my previous pregnancies. Every single morning, I would gag non-stop until I finally vomited. Not very fun when you're in a caravan. This was a pretty great thing for me, though. If I gagged or threw up every day, it gave me reassurance that in my belly I had a little clinger who was fighting to live. Fighting to be here. This statement couldn't be truer of our little miracle.

Given that I'm quite a big drinker, it wasn't hard for everyone to guess that I was once again pregnant. Everyone was so excited for us, but I, of course, was apprehensive. I was happy on the outside, but inside I was in constant fear. While we were away on holidays, I refused to have sex. I didn't want to risk any trauma to that vicinity, which Tommy completely respected. Towards the end of the trip, I can remember wiping after going to the toilet and having little specs of brown fleshy tissue on the toilet paper. Ah. Here we go.

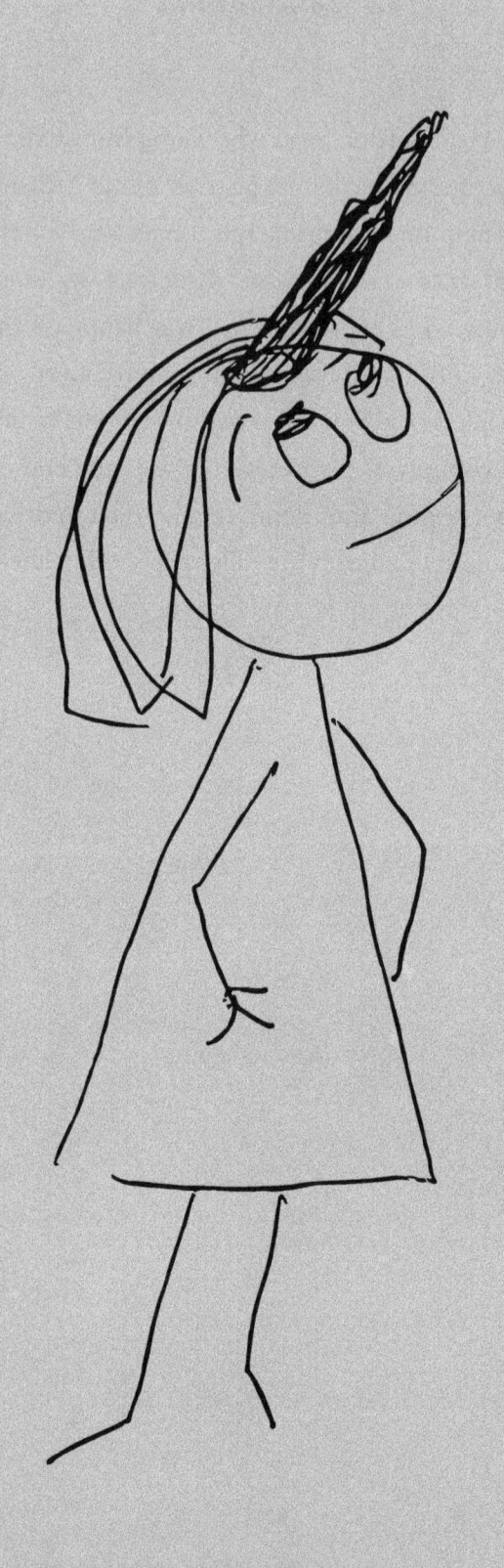

SUCH A UNICORN

WE RETURNED HOME from holidays, and I had had no bleeding, just a few specs of brown. I was still extremely sick every morning, which both Tommy and my mother reassured me was a great thing. It didn't settle my unease. I went to see my GP, who ordered bloods and an early dating scan for me. She told me I was to do no exercise or have sex whatsoever, until we reached the 12-week scan. On the morning of the early scan, I felt sick with anxiety. I didn't even want to go. I remember going to the toilet at work that morning and whether I had imagined it or not, I could have sworn there was pink discolouration on the toilet paper when I wiped. I mentioned this Tommy as we were headed to the scan and said, "Just be prepared for some not so good news." He rubbed my hand.

My name was called, and I realised the lady doing my scan was the one I had previously met who had also suffered a miscarriage. Thank God. I knew I was in safe hands and that she would keep me well informed for the duration of the scan. I emptied my bladder and we went straight for the internal scan. I felt sick. I was so nervous! In went the probe, and I desperately watched the screen.

"Look, there it is!" the sonographer exclaimed. "152 beats per minute. Look at it go! You're measuring 7 weeks 5 days."

I let out a little sigh of relief. So far, this baby had lived longer than my previous four, so I was feeling slightly positive; but we weren't out of the woods yet. There was no point in getting too excited. Tommy was thrilled and couldn't stop smiling at the screen. We got some printed pictures of our little peanut and went back to our day.

The 12-week scan arrived after what felt like a lifetime. I was still throwing up every single morning and was eating so much bread to try and settle the sick feeling in my stomach. I'm usually the person who prepares all their lunches for the week and absolutely loves food, so how no one at work noticed me getting a toasted sandwich every single morning and turning my nose up at different foods is beyond me. I had requested to book my scan in with the same sonographer again, as I loved her and I knew she would look after me.

On the morning of the scan, I got a phone call from Radiology advising that she was unwell, and I had been booked in with someone else. I had a major freak-out over this. Was this a sign? Did this mean I was going to go to my scan only to have someone not let me see the screen, and have yet another baby with no heartbeat? I was peaking. I rang Tommy and absolutely panicked down the phone to him. He was so supportive and reminded me that I had vomited that morning, so everything was obviously fine.

The poor woman who was doing my scan. I do feel bad for how I treated her. In saying that, her tact was a little off. She let me see the screen and as soon as I saw my baby moving around happily,

I relaxed. I couldn't believe it. It was so big! The heartbeat was still going strong, and developmentally the baby was ticking all the right boxes. Hooray!

The woman then asked me one of the stupidest questions. I had been going to the same radiology clinic for all my scans, so my history would have been right in front of her, and I had seen it was also noted on the referral form. She said, "Any abnormalities with your previous pregnancies?"

I stared at her, looked over at Tommy blankly, then looked back at her and said, "Well, I miscarried all three previous pregnancies, so yeah, I guess you could say there were abnormalities."

She obviously hadn't bothered to look at my file, nor read on my referral that I had had three previous pregnancies but nil gestation, meaning none of them were successful. Come on, love, even I knew that one. She apologised profusely and attempted to say that it wasn't noted. Whatever. I could see my baby and that's all that mattered.

We got some fantastic pictures. The baby was poking its little tongue in and out of its mouth, bouncing around, rolling over and doing all sorts. I could have sat there watching it all day. The sonographer took multiple photos and mentioned that she needed extra pictures of the placenta and cord insertion. I didn't take much notice because as far as I was concerned, everything was going swimmingly. Tommy and I left the appointment feeling extremely optimistic, and thrilled that we had finally made it to the 12-week mark. Go us!

The following day, I had my follow-up appointment with my GP to discuss where I would like to have my antenatal care. Dr D reviewed the report from the scan and calmly told me that a velamentous cord insertion had been identified.

"Okay. What does that mean?" I asked.

"Right now, it doesn't mean much. It will need to be reviewed at the 20-week scan, when we are able to get a better view of it. It just means that the cord hasn't inserted where it should have. I would recommend that you and your husband refrain from having sex until after the 20-week scan. You are also not to do any form of exercise."

Holy shit. What? After determining I would have my care through the public hospital, I left the appointment and called my mother. She would be able to explain to me what a velamentous cord insertion meant.

I remember Mum kind of changing her voice when I told her what was on the report. She switched from mum to midwife very quickly as she explained what it meant. She sounded concerned. Basically, the cord usually inserts somewhere in the middle of the placenta, whereas a velamentous cord insertion is where the umbilical cord inserts into the foetal membranes, leaving rather large blood vessels exposed. GREAT! Fun fact: a velamentous insertion occurs in approximately 1% of pregnancies. Of course I had one. Given my level of stress with this pregnancy already, I kind of didn't need this. Anyway, I took it in my stride and just decided to do as I was told and wait until the 20-week scan.

I was still extremely sick at this point, vomiting every single morning. However, I needed constant reassurance that everything was okay. I was so lucky that my mother had her own private midwifery practice which she ran from home, which meant I showed up, at a very minimum, once a week (sometimes it was every second day), just to listen to my baby's heartbeat. Every single time, my lovely mother obligingly let me hear my baby's heart pumping away via her doppler. I will be forever grateful for this. I can imagine she was probably thinking I was being a bit ridiculous, but she never questioned it or made me feel like I was letting my anxiety get the better of me. I totally was, but just hearing the beautiful sound of that heartbeat immediately put my mind at ease.

I can remember the exact moment I first felt that beautiful flutter of my baby moving. I was 16 weeks pregnant and still vomiting each morning, which was so glamorous but in a sick way I loved the reassurance. I was sitting at my desk at work, and after everything I had been through, I was probably freakishly sensitive to any sort of sensation in my belly. I felt that gentle fluttering and I can remember initially thinking, *That's weird, I've never felt that before.* Then it clicked. Holy shit! That's the baby! HIIIII BABY!!!!! It was the best feeling in the world. The next morning was my rostered day off, and I can vividly remember waking up to a rolling sensation across my belly.

"Good morning, baby," I remember saying out loud as I rubbed my belly. This was such a glorious feeling. Not quite glorious enough to ease my anxiety – I still ended up at Mum's place most afternoons to hear the heartbeat, and I still was not quite letting myself attach to this baby for constant fear that I wouldn't get my happy ending.

As bub grew, I came to feel it move more and more. By 18 weeks I had stopped vomiting every morning but was able to feel more and more movement. Part of me wants to believe that our baby knew how insecure I was, so it made me so unwell until it was confident enough that I could feel its movement. Who knows? Our next scan was fast approaching. I booked in with my preferred sonographer again, as I was most comfortable with her and asked Mum to come with us. I wanted to have her in the scan from a medical perspective, and also because sometimes I forget what I'm told.

For some reason, on the morning of the scan I was riddled with anxiety. I nearly cancelled the appointment. I can remember sitting in the toilets at work thinking, *I don't even want to fucking go to this thing. It's going to be bad news. I've stopped vomiting and I haven't even felt the baby move. It's dead, I just know it. Fuck me, I'm so sick of this.*

Quite seriously, I was spiralling. After telling myself to get over myself, I went back and sat at my desk and stared blankly at the screen. About 30 minutes before Tommy was due to pick me up for the scan, I copped an almighty boot in the belly. I suddenly got tears in my eyes and couldn't stop smiling to myself like a complete weirdo. It was as if my baby was like, "Oi, lady. You're an idiot and I'm still here!" I instantly relaxed and was excited to see this little thing that was determined to have its presence known.

My name was called for the appointment. The sonographer also knew my mother so she was very excited to see her and welcome her into the appointment as well. She immediately brought bub's heartbeat up so we could all relax. I loved that about her. Whilst identifying that my placenta was quite honestly EVERYWHERE – there were three parts to this damn thing – she also identified what is known as an amniotic sheet. An amniotic sheet is caused by the membranes folding over and attaching to scar tissue in the uterus. Given that I had had two previous D&Cs, it wasn't all that surprising that I had scar tissue. It was also identified that the placenta was completely covering my cervix, which is known as placenta previa. Another fun fact: an amniotic sheet occurs in one in every 200 pregnancies, and placenta previa occurs in approximately four in every

1000 pregnancies. Why the hell was I getting all of these rare things occurring in my pregnancy? For a very long time I have said that my life is Murphy's Law, but I have since changed my attitude and decided I'm just a friggen unicorn. Unique as fuck, and not necessarily in a good way.

We left the appointment and Mum was concerned. She said that we would wait for the report, and I would also be able to discuss it with my midwife that the hospital had assigned to me. Her name was Jen* and she was beautiful. The following day, I received a call from my GP's office; she had received a copy of the results of my scan and requested an urgent appointment with me. Shit. Tommy was unable to attend, so I asked my mother to come with me. When we got to the appointment, Dr D honestly scared the living shit out of me.

"You are not to be doing any exercise or having sex. The likelihood of your placenta moving up out of the way of the cervix is slim to none. It is covering the os (the opening in the lower part of the cervix between the uterus and vagina) completely, which means you are also at risk of rupture, so you are not to go camping or be anywhere far away from a hospital."

My head was spinning. After the appointment, Mum drove me back to work. I can't remember the exact conversation, but I remember crying as we drove back and sat in the carpark of my work building. Basically, this pregnancy had turned into something very scary where I could start bleeding at any moment, and I needed to prepare myself for an early delivery via cesarean. I was devastated.

After texting Tommy the details in short, I pulled myself together and went back to work, trying to pretend that everything was fine.

In all fairness, everything was fine. The baby was doing really well; I just had to be extra vigilant for quite a while, and I had another scan scheduled for approximately 32 weeks to check on the placenta. If I made it that far.

I was terrified. Terrified of losing my baby and terrified at having to deal with this as our reality. When Tommy arrived home from work that evening, I allowed myself to cry. I explained to him the seriousness of the situation and we made a plan that if I ever rang him, regardless of what he was doing, he needed to make sure he answered that damn phone in case it was an emergency. You could see the stress of the pregnancy was starting to take its toll on Tommy as well. He was losing patience with trying to remain positive. We had fought so hard just to get to this point. Why did it have to keep being an uphill battle for us?

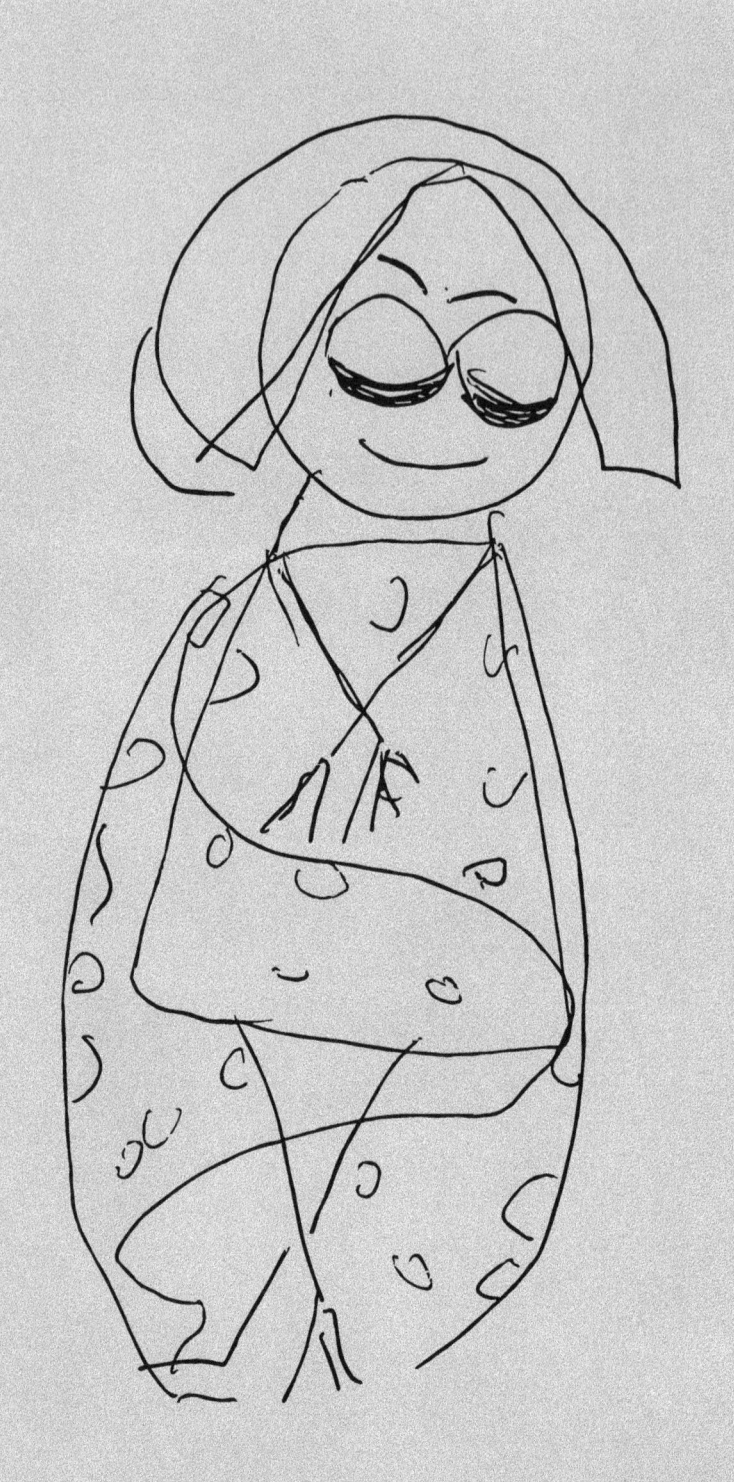

WRAPPED UP IN COTTON WOOL

THE NEXT TWELVE weeks passed in a bit of a blur. Everyone around me was on constant edge as to whether my placenta or velamentous cord would rupture. It was a long period of unease for everyone. At around the 28-week mark, Tommy and I had booked in for a Calmbirth class. For any first time parents or anyone who has had a particularly traumatic birth previously, I cannot recommend Calmbirth enough. It was upon completion of this course that I finally felt like I connected with my baby and accepted I was going to be a mother.

The course is an in-depth antenatal class that takes you through how to trust your body. It teaches you that your body already knows how to birth a baby without the assistance of any medical intervention. You do some hypnosis, which helps teach you breathing techniques to cope with labour, and most importantly, how to remain calm if things take a bit of a turn and you require medical intervention. It is mesmerising and very empowering. After the two-day course you leave feeling completely prepared and connected with your body, with so much confidence in your ability to birth your little one. Another major aspect of the course is to show your partner what a significant role they play in the birth. Tommy could not speak highly enough of the course and continues to encourage anyone expecting a baby to take part.

We were so happy that we had made it to 28 weeks without a bleed or any indication of a problem. We had four weeks to go before we had another scan and I had made a habit of saying out loud most days that "my placenta WILL move up and out of the way, and I WILL have a happy, healthy baby via vaginal birth". I may have sounded like a freak but hey, it made me feel better.

With the Calmbirth class, we were lucky enough that no other couple booked into the group session, and we ended up having a one-on-one with the instructor, in our own home. This instructor is hands down one of the most beautiful souls I have ever come across in my life. Her presence is so calming, and her own journey is far from one of pure bliss. I adore her. She is a midwife and also a paediatric nurse, so she has a wealth of knowledge and experience behind her. On the last day she decided to have a feel around and teach Tommy how to identify which part of the baby was where in my belly. She identified that bub was not yet head down, which isn't necessarily a bad thing, but she advised that I should be making sure I'm getting myself into certain positions so that bub was able to move into a better birthing position.

The instructor showed us some different baby spinning techniques which Tommy was able to help me with, and encouraged me to do some research on natural ways to help bub turn. I wasn't too concerned at this point. There was plenty of time for baby to turn, and we didn't know if I would even be able to birth naturally yet so it might not matter what position the baby was in. Given that we didn't know where the placenta was either, we were a bit reluctant to try anything too vigorous, and the instructor agreed. Tommy was so excited that when he felt around now, he could work out the spine, bottom and head of the baby. I think that helped him feel a bit more connected to the baby as well.

32 weeks arrived and off to the scan we went. Again, Mum came with us to make sure she took in any medical information that Tommy or I might miss. I had booked in with my preferred sonographer once again, and she called my name to come through. Straight away we saw the heartbeat pumping away nice and healthy. Thank God! Even more excitingly, the placenta had completely moved out of the way of my cervix. HOORAY!! My vision of vaginal birth was finally becoming a reality. Woohoo!

"So, bub is frank breech," the sonographer said. "Look at the little feet touching its forehead!"

What? I looked at Mum, confused, and her exacerbation was evident. "Oh my god, Fiona, if it's not one thing with you, it's another! We will have to start doing some serious baby spinning to get that baby's head down."

We got some fantastic photos of our baby at this scan. It was almost as though bub was staring straight at the screen for us. It was beautiful.

I was booked in for another scan at 36 weeks and an appointment was made with a highly recommended obstetrician at the hospital. My mother had worked with this doctor for quite some time, and I had heard a lot about him as he had been across all three of my previous miscarriages as well as every step of the way with my current pregnancy via my mother. I was excited to finally meet him. The appointment came and I was met with the biggest smile and a loud, booming voice. I loved him already! Dr E* is quite simply one of the most beautiful men I have had the pleasure of coming across on this earth. He truly listens to his patients' concerns or wants, and does everything in his power to support a natural birth for women. Many doctors could learn from this man, instead of telling women their pelvis is too small or that the baby won't fit, and they will need a C-section just because it suits them better. I'm not at all saying this is the case for all C-section births. I would like to hope that all C-sections happen for both the safety of the mother and baby. Unfortunately, I know this not to be true.

Dr E discussed with me the location of my placenta, which he was happy with. I raised my concerns with the amniotic sheet causing growth problems, and based on the frequent scans he advised that there seemed to be no evidence to show bub's growth was being hindered. Thank God. We discussed the position of the baby, and Dr E also had a feel around and confirmed it was still breech. He advised me that if bub was still frank breech at the 36-week scan, the option of having a manual turn, otherwise known as an ECV (external cephalic version), was available to me.

"I have a very high success rate with ECV. You are a first-time mother, which can make the turn a little difficult. However, you are not overweight, so it makes you a good candidate for success. You can think it over and we can discuss it further after the scan in four weeks if you like?" I felt so safe with him. "Now, are you having any bleeding after intercourse?" he asked.

"Huh? We were told we couldn't have sex because of the location of the placenta. Can we have sex?" I was flabbergasted. Tommy and I had basically gone eight months straight without sex, and now we were being told it was an option! Dr E looked at me and then looked at Tommy and started laughing. "Seriously, can we have sex?" I was almost begging.

Dr E looked pained and said, "Well, given that you haven't been having it, I would continue to do so until after the next scan. I'm sorry." He was genuinely sorry for both Tommy and me. Dammit!

The next four weeks were spent with me doing all sorts of "hippy shit", as Tommy so affectionately called it. He was very supportive of it, but that didn't stop him from making a little fun. I was getting regular acupuncture, burning moxa sticks on acupressure points on my toes, putting myself upside down on the couch, lying backwards on an ironing board, watching TV with my belly wedged into a donut floaty so I was on my belly, plus getting regular Bowen therapy from my mother. I did everything possible to help this baby turn head down.

I was feeling positive going into the 36-week scan. Even though I hadn't felt a major flip/movement of the baby, I felt confident that I had done everything I could. Once again, our favourite sonographer called our names in for our scan. The screen showed our baby, and lo and behold... it hadn't turned. Bub was still happily in the exact same position it had been in four weeks ago, and probably since 28 weeks when our Calmbirth instructor originally identified the position.

Great. Tommy and I had already discussed whether we would have an ECV if bub hadn't turned, so I knew this was our next step.

The following day we met with Dr E and agreed to have an ECV.

"I have a question to ask you," I said. Dr E turned his attention to me. "Next weekend is my grandmother's 80th birthday in Melbourne. I was overseas for her 70th, so I would really like to go to her 80th if I can. Are you able to give me a certificate to fly? I will have Mum with me the whole time and will make sure we know where a hospital is at all times in case something happens." I waited for his response. I would be 37 weeks pregnant at the time of flying, so I knew it would be a risk and there was a major possibility that I couldn't go. But I had to ask.

Dr E closed his eyes for a moment and then said, "That will be fine. I am happy for you to fly because your mother will be with you for the entire duration. We will book you in for ECV at 37+5 the week after, as long as nothing happens while you are away."

Phew! I was so excited. My grandmother didn't think I was going to be able to make it, so this would be a fantastic surprise for her.

We flew to Melbourne with my mother. Given how pregnant I was, I had to wear those super sexy deep vein thrombosis socks that legitimately went all the way up to my thighs and were held on over my giant belly by a belt. I felt so attractive. Not! My grandmother got the shock of her life when Tommy and I showed up at her party. It is a memory I will always cherish, and I am forever grateful that bub decided to play the game and not make an entrance while we were such a long way from home. We made the most of our time in this part of the country and visited the Twelve Apostles, and drove some of the Great Ocean Road. By the time we got home, I was tired and exhausted. Thank God I had finished work the week before and had one day to rest before the ECV was booked.

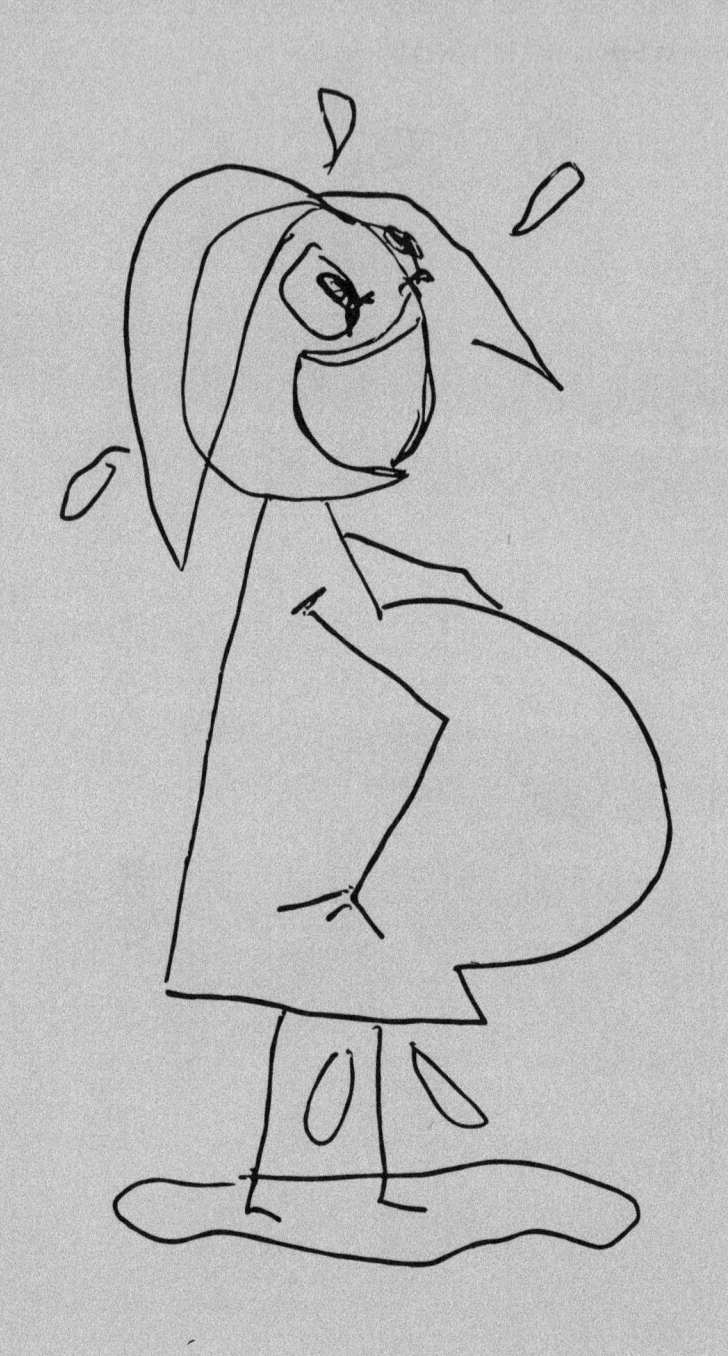

PREGNANCY GLAM

THE MORNING OF the ECV arrived, and I had this abnormal calm within me. I hadn't thought too much about it and I was keen to put some of my Calmbirth techniques into practice. I think the fact that I was so calm helped to keep Tommy calm about the situation too. Either that, or I was your typical first-time mum and kind of naïve slash a little stupid, and not really understanding the magnitude of the situation.

Looking back, I cannot stop laughing when I retell the story of my ECV. As per usual, not so funny in the moment but when you relive it, it's hysterical. We had packed a bag in preparation, as sometimes when an ECV is performed, the baby doesn't like it and an emergency C-section is required. Given I had a velamentous cord insertion, this was a high possibility; and let's face it, I was a unicorn. If anyone was going to have their ECV turn into an emergency C-section, it was me. Tommy and I met Mum on the maternity ward, and she came in with us. My midwife Jen was also there. For an ECV, the process is to begin by administering a drug via an IV to relax the uterus. The whole time, your baby's heartbeat is being monitored to ensure they are not in distress. I can't remember the exact time, but I feel it was about 30 minutes after the drug had been administered when Dr E came in, ready to perform the turn.

Now, my mother is usually a very calm human being when it comes to taking care of pregnant women. So many women have had her help while they birth their babies and even in the toughest of situations, she remains a calm voice of reason. In saying that, when she is anxious, I swear to God she makes the whole room feel it. Watching your daughter have an ECV performed by a colleague you hold in high regard, I can imagine, is a stressful point in your life. Anyway, Dr E came in, put a quick scan over my belly to have a look at the position of the baby, and then started rubbing moisturiser over my stomach. I was still very calm through all of this. I had this odd sense of "it's all going to be okay", so I wasn't too concerned.

The next steps happened extremely quickly. The room was completely silent as Dr E rubbed the lubricant all over my belly. He then said, "Okay, let's turn." He had barely finished this sentence before his hands dug deep into my belly and I had the air knocked out of me with pain.

All I can remember is hearing my mother scream, "Breathe, Fiona!" I tried desperately to get air into my lungs while my whole body was tensing, trying to fight what was happening. It was over as quickly as it started. 30 seconds max, I think. The room was still silent, Tommy was in shock over what had just happened, and Dr E had cream all over his hands and was desperately trying to get the scan to bring up the heartbeat.

"Where is the heartbeat?!" Mum was panicked. I could feel the baby moving, so at this point I started hysterically laughing like a full-on crazy person. I'm talking tears down my face kind of laughter. Poor Dr E had butterfingers with all the moisturiser on his hands, so the scanner was slipping all over the place. Finally, he got the heartbeat; bub was head down and in absolutely no distress.

"There it is," he breathed. "Head is down, and the heartbeat is good." I could see he was visibly shaking. Keep in mind that I'm still giggling like a freak here and Tommy is just staring around at everyone in shock and confusion. Next thing, Dr E shook his head vigorously and blew out a loud sigh of relief with his lips flapping together like a horse. Well, this just tipped me over the edge. Again, I was pissing myself laughing.

The tension in the room had eased and then my mother, bless her, announced, "I brought some choc chip caramel slice! Does anyone want some slice?" Seriously. Who brings slice to something like this?

Dr E was so relieved, and he and my mother discussed how nervous they were for each other over a piece of choc chip caramel slice. It is an absolute honour to be asked to care for someone's family; Dr E did not want to have a failed ECV, and Mum didn't want me to be one of the few where the turn was unsuccessful. They were both relieved it had been a success and Dr E took a few extra bits of the slice Mum had baked, and continued on his rounds. I remained for a further 20 minutes of monitoring to make sure bub was okay and we were then sent on our merry way.

That afternoon I did my best to concentrate on feeling bub's movements. Given the change in position, I felt confused as to where I was feeling movement. The important thing was that I was still feeling plenty of movement. Mum was continuously texting me to make sure I was okay. I was sore, and my belly was bleeding a little from fingernail scratches, but otherwise I was fine. I spent the afternoon napping and just enjoying having Tommy home for the day.

The following morning Tommy left for work early. I lay in bed for a while holding my belly and concentrating on movement. I felt bruised. The bottom of my abdomen felt too damn sore even for the blankets to be touching it. Then as I got up out of bed, I felt fluid in my underwear. Ew. Had I just peed a little? Come on, girlfriend, get your shit together.

I went to the toilet and noticed a smell almost similar to semen. Knowing damn well we hadn't had sex, I didn't think much of it and continued about my day. I had agreed to go in to see Mum that morning for a Bowen therapy session and I was getting my hair done at lunch. I went to Mum's house, and she performed some Bowen therapy on me. It was so relaxing. She asked how I was feeling and if I'd had much movement since the turn.

"I'm confused about the movement," I said. "I was so used to feeling it at the top of my belly, but now it's almost like I have to concentrate to feel the movement. How about I think I pissed myself a bit this morning? Pregnancy is so glam." I'm very open with my mother, so I figured she'd get a giggle out of it.

Instead, she was more questioning. "Was it actually wee? Or did it have a smell sort of like semen?" she asked. How did she know?

"It did, actually! How did you know that?"

"It sounds like you've had a hind-leak. Some amniotic fluid has escaped. No contractions? Even when you're expressing colostrum?" She had gone full midwife mode on me. I hadn't had any contractions whatsoever. "Okay," she said. "If you have any more leaking, you will need to contact Jen and let her know. Sometimes after an ECV it can cause a leak from the pressure of the turn."

I felt fine, so again, I didn't think much of it. I was tired though. I left my mother's house and went to the hairdresser. After nearly falling asleep in the chair, I knew my day was over and I just wanted to go straight home to bed. I was absolutely shattered. And every movement felt painful after having the turn the day before. I knew I needed rest. I cranked up the aircon when I got home and lay down for a sleep.

About half an hour after I lay down, I suddenly felt a gushing sensation. I leapt out of bed and raced to the toilet. This didn't feel like wee, and I had absolutely no control over it. It smelt as though a bucket of semen had fallen out of me. Hmm, another hind-leak, I suspected. Although it was a hell of a lot. As I wiped and stood up to go to the bathroom, I was still dripping.

I remember saying out loud, "Fucking yuck, man."

I grabbed my phone and sat back on the toilet because I continued to leak. Attractive, I know. I dialled Jen's number.

"Hi, Jen. So, I just thought I should let you know I had a bit of a leak this morning. And I've just had a massive gush of fluid. Is that normal?"

Jen listened intently on the other end of the phone. "Well, it sounds like your waters have broken. How exciting! Why don't you come up to the hospital and we'll check everything out and make sure your waters have definitely broken and go from there."

Huh? Holy shit. "Oh, really?" I said stupidly. "Okay. Um. Well, Tommy doesn't finish work for another hour so is it okay if we come up after that?" I needed to pack my bag, express some more colostrum, and get my head around the fact I was having a friggen baby.

"That's fine. Just send me a text when you're on your way up and I'll meet you on the ward." Jen hung up the phone.

I didn't call Tommy because I knew he'd freak out and leave work early when there really wasn't any need.

I called my mother, who answered knowing full well I'd had a leak that morning.

"Hello?" she said. "I'm just with a patient – is everything okay?"

Suddenly I turned into a freaking child and my voice shook down the phone as though I was about to cry.

"My waters broke." What the hell was happening? I was legitimately on the verge of tears.

"Okay, have you called Jen?" Mum was trying to remain professional in front of her client. I managed to squeak a yes. "I'll call you back once I've finished this appointment." And Mum hung up.

Right, Fiona, grab your lady balls and sort your shit out here. I grabbed some towels because yep, I was still dripping. I laid a path from the toilet to the bathroom, where I had my syringes for expressing colostrum. I stood in the bathroom over towels and hand-expressed some colostrum with no pants on, just casually leaking onto the pile of towels. As I said, pregnancy is such a glamorous business.

2.30 pm rolled around and I knew Tommy would be finished work. He sent me a message saying he had finished, so I called him.

"Hey, babe?" he answered.

I tried to be as calm and breezy as possible. For anyone that knows me, I am not breezy. "Heyyyyyy. So, are you coming straight home or are you going somewhere beforehand?" I asked.

"Straight home. Why, what's wrong?" He sounded concerned.

"Oh. Um. Well... my waters broke." Like I said, I am not breezy. But I try really hard.

"Did they?" he was so excited. "I knew something was going on by your voice. We're having a baby! I'll be home soon. Do we need to go to the hospital?"

I explained what Jen had said, and that because there was some pinkish fluid in amongst my waters I needed to get checked out and see if I was having any contractions. By the time Tommy got home I was ready to go. He had a quick shower just in case we were at the hospital all night, and we made our way back into town.

Jen met us on maternity ward. I had put a pad in my underwear to catch what was STILL leaking. Jen asked me to change it and hand her the used pad so she could determine if it was in fact amniotic fluid. I went to the bathroom and changed my pad. I looked down and saw a rank gloopy stringy chunk hanging out. "Fuck, this is gross," I can remember thinking. I later realised this was the mucus plug. But again, it's rank. Jen assessed the pad and confirmed it was amniotic fluid.

I was dilated 1cm and having no contractions. Given everything was fine with bub, I was free to go home. Now, when your waters break, you are at risk of infection. The doctors on the ward wanted me to have antibiotics at this point, which I declined. I didn't see the point in unnecessarily having antibiotics when no infection was present. I'm also not an idiot and would never put my unborn child at risk, but taking antibiotics "just in case" wasn't really my jam. Jen took a swab of my cervix to be sent away for testing, and I was to come back the following morning for another check-up unless I went into labour beforehand.

We got home early in the evening and were both on edge, just waiting for it to happen. I wasn't feeling anything, though. Neither of us got much sleep that night. We were both tossing and turning, waiting to be woken up by contractions that never came.

The following morning, we tiredly made our way up to the hospital for an 8am appointment. I asked my mother to meet us up there as I had a feeling the doctors would push me into doing something I didn't want to do, so I wanted a voice of medical reason there for me just in case. I was taken into a room and bub was monitored – heartbeat was happy, and no contractions were present. Great.

The results for my swab hadn't yet returned, and in came the on-call doctor again wanting to push antibiotics into me "just in case". Call me crazy, but I know what antibiotics do to my gut, so I didn't want to have the first thing my baby had in their gut be antibiotics unless it was genuinely needed. Of course, the doctor made me feel horrible, as though I was putting my baby at unnecessary risk. I felt like telling her to fuck right off. I understand you are just doing your job, but I'm not an idiot. I had done my research and I knew that I didn't NEED antibiotics unless an infection had been detected.

"If the swab comes back positive for an infection, then of course I will have antibiotics," I said. "But I do not feel the need to have them unless there is a proven reason." I was trying to be direct without telling the woman where to shove it.

After the doctor finally left me alone, Jen asked me what I wanted to do. "We can induce you now that you're here, or you can wait until labour starts. We should get the results of the swab back in the morning, so you'll most likely have to come back tomorrow even if you haven't gone into labour, as we'll need to continue to swab for infection because the longer you go with broken waters, the more likely an infection is." She was so nice with her delivery. "I'll give you guys some time to think about what you want to do."

I sat on the bed, listening to my baby's heartbeat ticking away and just stared at the ceiling for a minute. This isn't how it was supposed to happen. My waters were meant to break, and I was meant to go into spontaneous labour. I closed my eyes for a second while Tommy and Mum spoke to each other quietly. I could feel myself about to cry. I had gotten so far in this pregnancy, managing to avoid rupture or an early C-section, and having a successful turn. Why had the brakes hit at this crucial moment? I didn't want to be induced. But at the same time, I had this sickening feeling in the pit of my stomach that the longer I left my waters broken, the more risk I was posing to my baby, and I didn't want to get this far only for something fatal to happen just because I didn't want to be induced.

With tears in my eyes, I said to Tommy and my mother, "I think we should get induced in the morning. I can't keep waiting for this to happen and worrying about losing this baby when we've come so close. It's not what I wanted or how I pictured it, but I think it's the right thing to do."

Jen came back into the room, and we explained our plans. She booked us in for induction at 6am on Sunday the 11th of November 2018. Remembrance Day. We felt like it was a good sign.

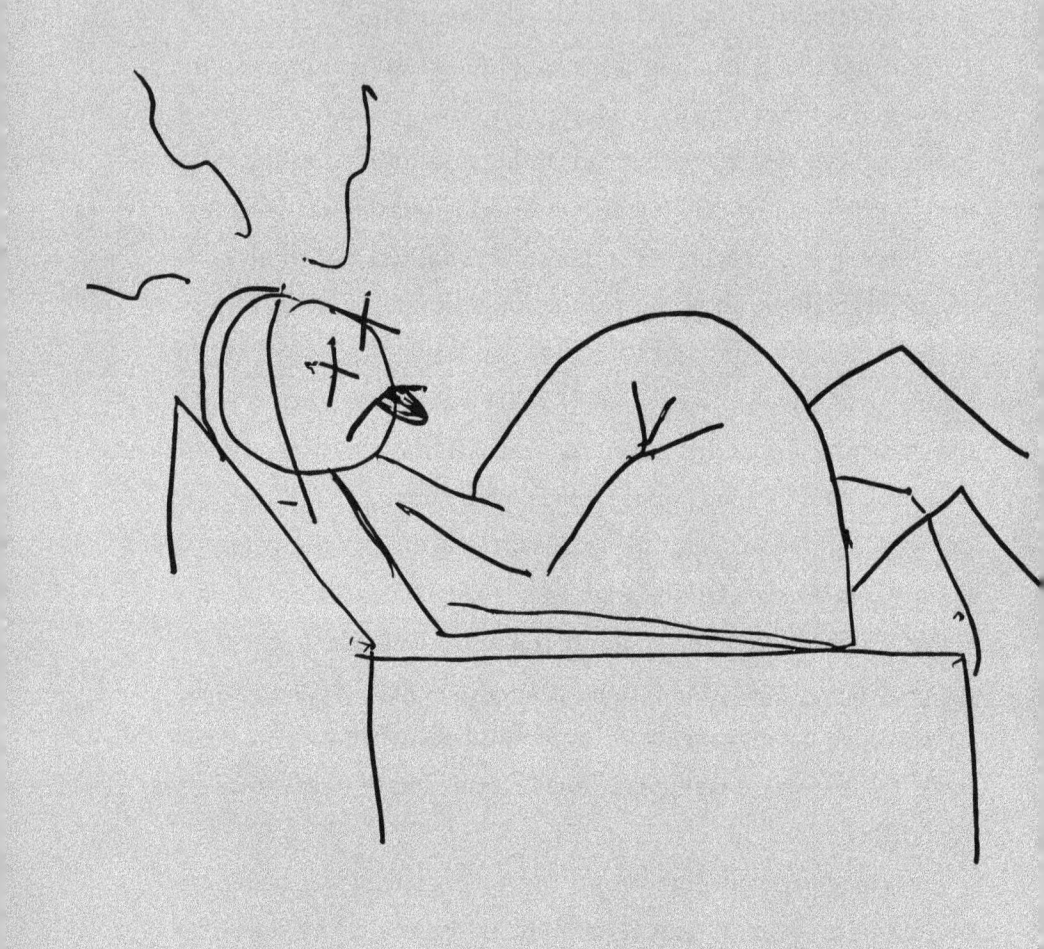

A DAY (OR TWO) TO REMEMBER

WE GOT HOME mid-morning and both tried to have a sleep. We had read that clary sage was a powerful essential oil in bringing on labour. The small bottle said to put no more than four drops in the diffuser. I pumped about 20 in there and lay down beside it. I couldn't sleep. Neither could Tommy. Our heads were spinning and we were feeling a little defeated. We decided that we would spend the afternoon doing some relaxation and some acupressure on me to try and help labour happen naturally. With every acupressure point, Tommy applied a stupid amount of clary sage to the spot as well. Honestly, we used over half a bottle. It was a little extreme to say the least.

I wanted to feel better, so I suggested we went to the nearby pub for dinner with his parents. It was going to be the last time we would be going out without a baby, so I put some make-up on, did my hair nicely, and stinking of clary sage we went for dinner. It was at dinner that I first noticed contractions. I didn't say anything to Tommy because I didn't want to scare the contractions away. So I just kept quiet. I think he knew something was up, though, because I was very quiet. Gradually they grew but again, I didn't want to scare them away. I ate my dinner and was absolutely knackered. I knew I needed to sleep before the induction in the morning, so we went home. We were in bed relatively early, and I heard Tommy start to snore shortly after we flicked off the lights.

The first contraction to wake me was at approximately 10:40pm. I put my calm birthing techniques into practice and breathed my way through it. I fell asleep shortly after. This carried on until about 3:00am, by which time they had ramped up quite a lot. I woke Tommy as I decided I needed some support in keeping me calm. The poor bloke flew out of bed, turned on all the lights and started playing music to try and keep the ambience going. Bless him. I texted Jen to say that my contractions had started, and we would no longer need to be induced. Thank God! I also texted my mother the same, as she was going to be at the hospital for us as well.

By about 6am my contractions had almost disappeared. They were still happening, but it felt like they were getting easier, not harder. Mum suggested we both lie down and try to get some sleep, and she said she would come out later in the morning to check on my progress. We both had a bit of a snooze and not long into the nap I was woken with full-on contractions again. Phew! I was worried we had scared them away. We kept the clary sage pumping through the house in the hopes to keep the labour happening. Honestly, I'll be glad if I never smell that shit again. The amount we had flying around the place, it was potent.

I don't know about other mums but for me, I felt the need to squat every time I had a contraction. Given that I hadn't done any exercise for an entire nine months, my legs were already sore, but my body naturally just told me to do it, so I pushed through. By about 10 or 11 am, Mum arrived and listened to bub's heart. Everything was going smoothly, and my contractions were slowly increasing.

"Okay, you might want to think about driving into town. Whenever I have helped mothers birth and they live far away from the hospital, they've always said the worst part was the drive into town. You can continue labouring at my place until it's time." I was so grateful for my mother's experience. We lived approximately 40 minutes from the hospital, and Mum's house was just around the corner from it.

That drive into town was hands down awful. I was hunched over the backseat trying to tell myself to breathe; but I was so uncomfortable not being able to squat with every contraction that it was so difficult to even talk. Tommy kept talking and telling me to breathe and what a great job I was doing. He had the occasional "get the fuck out of the way, mate!" whilst driving, which is pretty funny now, but at the time I was feeling the same way. We finally arrived at my mother's house just as another contraction hit. I was pinned to the back seat holding onto it and breathing as deeply as I could until it passed. In the short time between contractions, I raced upstairs to the dark, airconditioned room Mum had ready for us, and lay down. I needed to sleep between them.

The female body is an incredible thing. Somehow, I was able to fall into the deepest sleep in between each contraction, throw myself up over the side of the bed once I felt one starting, begin my squat until it had passed, and then lie back down again and fall asleep. Insane!

Couldn't do that now if I tried. After a while I felt I needed hot water on my back; Tommy and I relocated to the shower, where I sat on the yoga ball with boiling hot water pounding my back and squatting over the ball every time a contraction hit. Tommy was fantastic. I honestly couldn't have asked for a better birthing partner. The poor bloke had a runny nose and a bit of a flu, but he never left my side the entire time, and for that I am so thankful.

At around 1.30pm my breathing and noises started to change. As the contractions became closer together, with every squat and breath I took it was starting to sound almost like a bit of a grunt. Mum gently came into the room and said, "It's time." Between contractions, we bundled me back into that godforsaken car and made the two-minute drive to the hospital. Again, probably the worst part of the entire experience. The car is not a comfortable place to have contractions, let alone in the peak of summer. We arrived at the hospital and parked nice and close. Between the car and getting into the birthing suite, I had to stop six times for contractions. I was so hot that I needed a shower to cool down; the air-conditioning in the hospital didn't even feel like it was on. It was, by the way; I just couldn't feel it.

Jen met us in the birthing suite, and we got straight in the shower. I was completely naked by this point and couldn't have cared less; I was overheating, and I could feel it. The swab test for the infection had returned and it had come back negative. Phew! No antibiotics. While I continued to squat in the shower with Tommy holding me and squatting along with me, Jen hooked me up to the CTG (cardiotocography) machine to monitor bub's heartbeat and also monitor my own.

"Fiona, your heartrate is up really high, which is the first sign of infection. Now, I know the swab came back negative, but if your heartrate doesn't go down, we're going to need to give you antibiotics," Jen said gently.

I shook my head vigorously. No. I didn't want this. Now, I am a very pale redhead who does not do well in heat at the best of times. Take into consideration that I was heavily pregnant, labouring, and had just walked through 50-thousand-degree heat and was already trying to cool myself down in the shower. Of course my heartrate was through the roof. I was hot and bothered!

My mum was in the room, as an additional support person only. However, having been a midwife for over 30 years, her wealth of experience couldn't be kept in at this point. I heard her gently say, "She has had a high heart rate throughout the entire pregnancy, and she has just walked up here in the heat whilst labouring. Maybe give her half an hour to cool down before you make a decision."

Jen agreed and went to add something to my chart. My mum then quietly said to me, "Fiona. Breathe. Get that heart rate down. I know you're hot, but you need to relax and cool yourself down or else you're going to have to have antibiotics."

Thankfully, I managed to cool down and bring my heartrate back into a satisfactory range. There was no need for antibiotics yet. We continued to labour in the shower for quite some time, until I decided I wanted to get in the bath. Being in the water was so relaxing and took all the weight of my belly off my back, and I could just rock on my hands and knees.

I remained in the bath for quite some time and began to feel the urge to push. I can remember it still being daylight outside, but

I have no idea what time this was. My body was telling me to push and push hard. I was on my hands and knees and taking massive deep breaths and pushing with everything I had. This went on for a while; a mirror was slid underneath me so Jen could see the baby's head. It was right there. Hearing her tell me she could see the baby's head, hearing my mother say, "Listen to your body," and Tommy say, "You're doing it, babe – we're going to meet our baby soon," encouraged me to keep pushing. I wanted to meet this baby so badly.

Jen then said to me, "Fiona, are you able to get out of the bath?"

I had dreamt of a water birth. So, there was no way I was getting out of here. "No," I simply said.

She knew I had wanted a water birth, but they have a duty of care to try and get you to a safer place to birth; however, they cannot force you mid-labour unless there is a danger to you or the baby.

"Tommy, can you come and stand around here. I'm going to get Fiona to sit back and when the baby comes out, I'm going to hand it straight to you to catch, okay?"

I can remember this moment vividly. It was about to happen! I had been on my hands and knees this entire time, and it was now time to roll back and hold my knees up and push for the last few times. As I pushed myself back in the water and was on my back, I suddenly felt agony. I cried out in pain.

"No!" I yelled. "No, I can't be on my back!"

The pain in my lower back was too much to bear. I needed the weight off it, so I went back to my hands and knees. By this time, it was dark. I had been pushing for what seemed like an eternity and still had no baby. The baby's heartrate was doing well so no concern there; but why hadn't I gotten this thing out yet?

"Fiona, you've been pushing for about an hour now and we haven't progressed very far. I'm going to need you to roll over so I can do an internal assessment to see what's going on." Jen was talking quietly to me.

Shit. I didn't want to go on my back. I ended up kind of on my side with one leg out of the bath so she could have a look. I remember Tommy talking to me, telling me how well I was doing, but I knew something was wrong.

"Yep. Okay. We have about 2cm of cervix pinched down under the baby's head. You're only about 8 cm dilated and the rest is pinched. We're going to have to get some gas in here for you, and you can't push any more until we can get the rest of your cervix dilated around the baby's head."

Panic. 8cm! This was bullshit. Why had my body told me to push so early if I wasn't even already dilated properly? At this moment I felt my body change. Fear set in. I didn't know what was going on or why this was happening.

Let me just say that trying not to push while you're contracting is damn near impossible. Your whole body is basically forcing you to push whether you want to or not, and trying to breathe through that is extremely difficult. I can remember my mother telling me not to push and almost yelling at me to breathe. Finally, the gas was wheeled in, and I took in five enormous breaths of it. Ahhhhhhhhhhhhhhhhh. I immediately started hallucinating and imagining that my mother was paying me out. So I mouthed off at her for being ever so subtle in an extremely sarcastic manner. She hadn't said a thing, but in my head she had. I can remember Tommy pissing himself laughing that I had suddenly piped up and mouthed off at my mother for no apparent reason after I had basically been mute for so long. Damn, another contraction; I sucked in a huge, deep breath of gas, trying not to push. My whole body was convulsing in an effort not to push.

The next few hours are a massive blur to me. I have flashbacks of some not-so-pleasant moments, but from what I've been told, we moved from the bath to lying in the shower while I hung off the gas. Tommy apparently lay down beside me on the floor of the shower, gently telling me to breathe through it all. We then moved to the bed, where I was on all fours and had Mum, Jen and Tommy pressing down extremely hard on different acupressure points every time a contraction came. I remember being back in the bath and having a doctor standing over me saying something along the lines of, "This is going to end in caesarean, and I'm about to leave for the night; so either we go now, or you have to wait for me to come back once I get the call."

I was still sucking gas and shaking my head so hard. No! I had come so far. Let me keep going. I was fine. I could get this baby out. I just needed time. But of course, I couldn't speak. My beautiful husband, who was holding the back of my head while I sobbed into his chest shaking my head, calmly said to the rude doctor, "Well, mate, I think we just need a bit more time." And with that he left. Call me crazy, but women are extremely vulnerable while they are birthing. Don't be a cock and stand over a naked woman dictating what is going to happen to her. If I wasn't incapable of speaking at this point, I would have told him to fuck right off.

The on-call consultant was a small woman who I feel was useless. Hours later she came in to do an internal assessment. This, by far, was the most painful internal I have ever experienced. And I have had a lot. I still have flashbacks of trying to kick this woman away from me. She was aggressively pushing my cervix back, trying to stretch it over the baby's head, which was still presenting at this point.

"It's brow presentation. You're going to need a C-section."

After she left, I needed to get off my back. It was agony. Back on my hands and knees, I was still trying not to push. Little did I know at this point, but my mother had said to Jen, "I think you're going to need an epidural." Prior to the birth, I had expressed my wishes for a natural birth free from medication or an epidural unless absolutely necessary, and I knew my mother fully supported me in that.

"Fiona, I know it's not what you want, but we're going to need to get you an epidural to try and help you relax and get that cervix to finish dilating. You won't be able to feel the contractions, so your body won't force you to push, okay?" Jen said to me.

"Yes! Please! Mum, please let me have the epidural!" In my head I said this because I knew she would fight for me to have the birth I wanted. In no way did I think she would prevent me from having medication or the epidural, which is how it came across.

"I won't stop you from having the epidural, Fiona; I think you need it," she calmly said. I couldn't explain to her what I meant. I was in so much pain and trying not to push.

As I said, I was out of it at this point. Poor Tommy. He was extremely sleep-deprived and quite sick. I didn't know that he and Mum had been tag teaming to take short breaks to regather themselves and wipe away their tears, so that I was never alone. When you're the one birthing, you honestly do not take into consideration what it must be like to watch someone you love in so much pain.

From what Tommy tells me, the anaesthetist who came to give me the epidural had just returned from a big holiday in Thailand,

and it was his first shift back. When trying to put fluid in this giant needle, he dropped the bag and bent the entire needle. He then proceeded to try and straighten the needle so it could be used, all while Tommy was watching and getting more and more horrified that this big bent needle was about to go into his wife's spine.

"How about I just take this one and give you a new one?" Thankfully, Jen had been watching as well and took a bit of control of the situation.

"Okay, Fiona, I am going to put the needle in your back now, so I just need you to hold still," the anaesthetist said to me.

Hold still? Yeah. Okay, buddy. He waited until a contraction had passed and I sat as still as I possibly could. To be honest, I didn't even feel the needle. Thankfully, it was a fantastic epidural and immediately I started to get less and less feeling in my lower body.

By the time the epidural had completely kicked in, it was after midnight. I was able to finally talk and tell Tommy that I was okay. I apologised to Mum for mouthing off to her earlier in the evening, and explained what I had meant when I begged her to let me have the epidural.

Unfortunately, Jen had worked over her time limit so she had to leave. She told me what an amazing job I had done, and she knew I would get through fine. She handed me over to another midwife who was just beautiful, although I can't remember her name. Through an IV, syntocinon was administered to help induce me further and encourage my cervix to finish dilating. In the meantime, the staff wheeled a bed in for Tommy and told us both to get some sleep.

Tommy went to wash his face and while he did so, Mum sat beside me telling me not to give up. I was exhausted.

"I'm not going to give up yet. As long as the baby is happy, I'll get it out," I said to Mum. I didn't know she had been communicating with Dr E via text all night, as unfortunately he was not on call that weekend. However, he was desperate to hear how I was going and had apparently kept offering to come in to assist if required. At this point, it was unnecessary. I was still pushing so well that Mum had complete faith I would get the baby out without requiring a C-section. After Tommy had freshened up, Mum let us be and he crawled into the bed with me.

He silently wept into my neck, and he cuddled me and I kept whispering, "I'm okay. I know it doesn't seem like it while I'm in the midst of labour, but I promise you I'm okay." He lay with me for about half an hour, told me he loved me, and crawled into the bed that had been brought in for him. We both needed the rest.

After about two hours of sleep, Mum woke me up and said, "Okay, Fiona, we're going to bring you out of the epidural, and you need to start pushing again. We'll give you a minute to wake up, and then we'll help you into position, as you're probably going to find it tough to feel your legs."

Mum gently woke Tommy up as well. By this point it was about 2.30am, I think. In a daze, Tommy crouched over on all fours with his head in the pillow, half asleep. He is a terrible sleepwalker, so I think for a while he didn't realise he was half awake. He stayed in that position for about ten minutes before Mum again tapped him and told him to go wash his face and wake up, because I needed him. He did as he was told in his sleepy state.

This is where it got really fun. Note the sarcasm. I still couldn't feel my legs, but going from zero contractions to full blown 10 cm dilated ready-to-pop-this-thing-out contractions isn't really a pleasant time, let me tell you. As I came out of the epidural, I needed to get off my back; the agony and pain in my spine was too much in that position. Having been shoved straight back into my labouring trance, I managed to tell everyone I wanted to be on my hands and knees. The new midwife, Tommy and Mum all swivelled me around and shoved my knees up underneath me as I still couldn't feel my legs, and again, I started pushing. Things get slightly blurry for me here. From memory, I had the midwife pushing down on my perineum because it gave me a sense of where I needed to push. Keep in mind that the epidural was still wearing off so all I could feel were the contractions. This went on for some time – what felt like a lifetime again. Everyone could see the baby's head, and I was pushing with everything I had, so why wasn't this thing coming out? I can legitimately remember thinking, "Every other fucking woman gets these things out, why can't I? Push harder!" I was determined to get the baby out.

It is crucial to try and keep moving during labour. The slightest movement can open your hips just that little bit more and allow the baby to get out. The midwife suggested I try going on my back again, with my legs up in stirrups. I nodded, as my hands and knees clearly weren't working. The three of them flipped me over and put my legs up in the stirrups. I could feel everything by this point. As soon as my legs were up in the stirrups and I was flat on my back, I began screaming. Full-blown screaming. "My back! No!" I was in absolute agony. I was desperately trying to kick off the stirrups, despite my legs still being quite numb, just to get off my back.

"I think we're spine on spine," I heard Mum say.

I got myself over onto my side and forced myself back into a hands and knees position. I was not going onto my back again.

While I did this, I didn't notice Mum leave the room. I had my head leaning on Tommy's forehead, and this was the first time I remember saying, "I can't do it. I can't do it anymore." I was crying, defeated.

"It's okay, babe. We can see the head. You've nearly got our baby out." I could feel Tommy's tears as well. It was horrible for him to watch me in so much pain.

Then Mum leaned over and said, "Fiona. Dr E is going to come in to see what needs to happen. Don't you give up yet. He said not to give up! He might be able to help get the baby out. Otherwise, he will take you down to theatre for a caesarean, okay? But you need to be ready to push. We'll put the epidural back up to give you some pain relief."

I nodded, not able to speak through tears. I hadn't realised that the epidural was on a drip that had a button you could pump the fluid into me with. Tommy was in control of the button by this point, but you could only press it once every 15 minutes or so. The first few presses took the edge off for me and I was able to communicate.

"Oh, you bastards have been holding out on me, hey? Pump that shit up, dude!" I said to everyone in the room. Tommy laughed and I think it was a relief to everyone that I was okay. As soon as the machine beeped that enough time had passed, Tommy kept pressing that button for me, bless him. He was done with seeing me in pain.

Mum again said to me, "Dr E will be here in a minute, but don't give up, Fiona. You're so close!"

The stupid consultant who had earlier given me the roughest internal ever was again in the room. "It's brow presentation. Dr E will need to do a caesarean, I've already told you this," she stated. Brow presentation means that the baby has its eyebrows presenting, and it's damn near impossible to get the baby out.

At approximately 4.45am, Dr E walked in. I felt a huge sigh of relief when I saw that big, beautiful smile, and a huge ball rose in my throat. He did such a gentle internal assessment, got an ultrasound machine so he could see the definitive position the baby was in, and professionally put that mole of a consultant in her place. "The baby is occiput posterior presentation, not brow. If it was brow, it would not have made it this far down into the pelvis," Dr E stated. Basically, the baby had gotten itself spine on spine, which is why I was in excruciating pain whenever I was on my back; and the part of its head that was presenting was pretty much its entire forehead just above the brow line. So, with every single push, the baby's neck was extending further back as though looking up at the sky; but when they are spine to belly, their chin can tuck up under their neck to make a clean exit. Not a fun time for me or the baby.

Given that bub's heart rate was monitored the entire time and it was still quite happy where it was, and the fact that I was pushing fine, Dr E said to me, "Fiona, I'm just going to do another quick internal and then we are going to try with a suction cap if I can get it over the baby's head, okay?"

I nodded. Do what you gotta do, man. After a quick internal, he told us that the suction cap would just slip off, so he would have to use forceps and carry out an episiotomy. I had heard my mother speak of forceps deliveries and they were not pleasant to watch. Even as a midwife today, she cannot watch a forceps delivery, and chooses instead to stay up with the mother as an encouraging voice. My legs were put up into stirrups and a shield was placed across my belly so that I couldn't see. I can remember my mother saying, "Tommy, don't watch! Focus on Fiona. They both came up with me as I closed my eyes in preparation to push.

"Okay, Fiona," I heard Dr E say, "nice big push for me." I took a deep breath and pushed with everything I had. "Excellent, nice work. Next contraction I want one more big push, okay?" Dr E was so encouraging. Both Mum and Tommy were holding onto me at this point, also encouraging me.

"Here comes the next contraction, Fiona. This is it, you're about to bring your baby into the world," I heard my mother say.

Again, I closed my eyes and drew in the biggest breath I possibly could, and then pushed with every ounce of energy I had left.

"Oh my god, look how tiny it is!" I heard my mother exclaim. I had a baby on my chest and it was crying. Thank fuck that was over.

"You did it, babe. Oh my god, you did it!" Tommy was kissing my forehead.

"Time of birth, 5.12am Monday 12th November," I heard Dr E say.

I felt instant relief. It was over. We finally had our little miracle.

"We don't even know if it's a boy or a girl yet. Are you going to look, Tommy?" my mother asked excitedly.

Tommy lifted one leg of the baby. "It's a girl. We had a girl!"

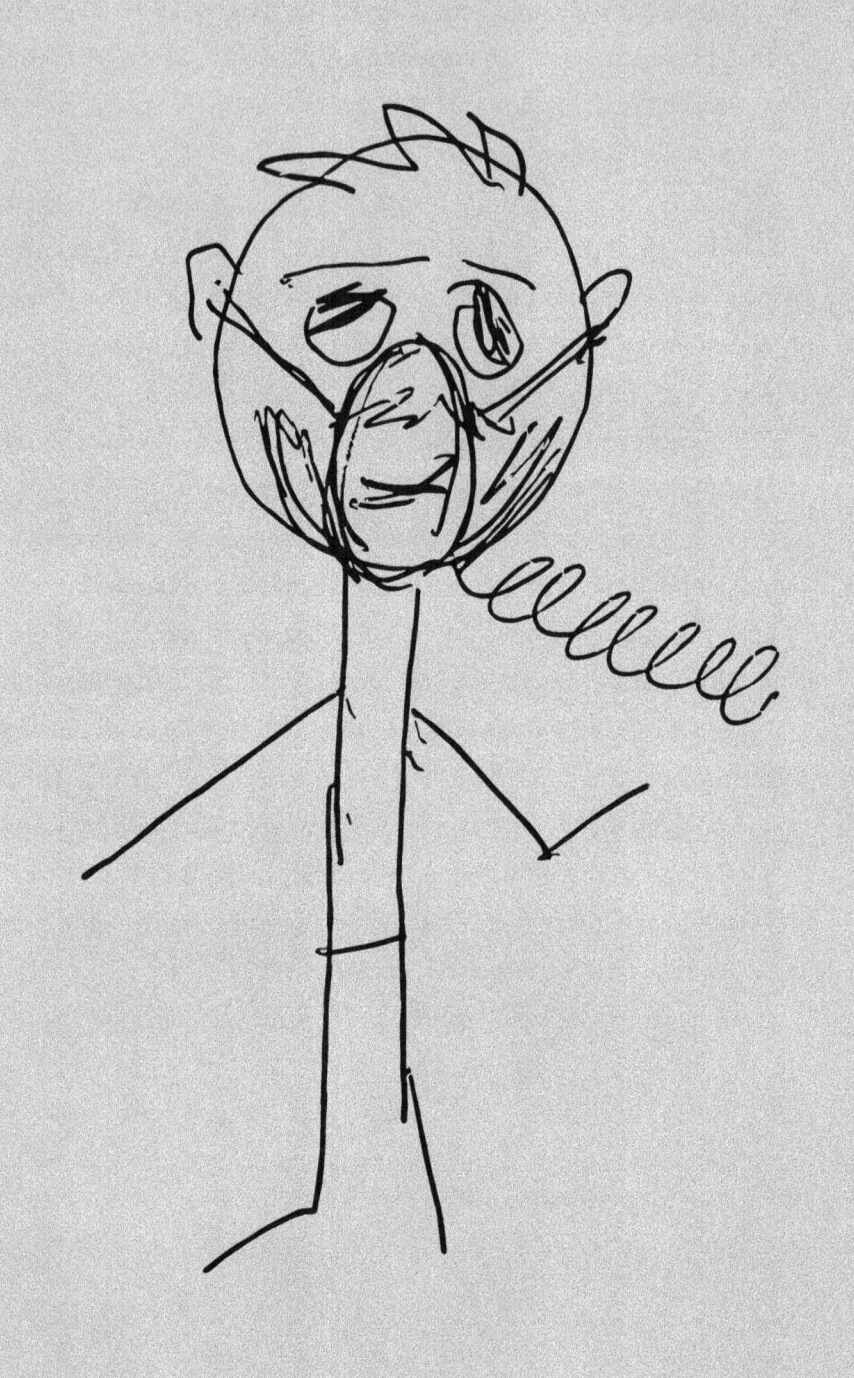

POST-BIRTH LOVE BUBBLE

AFTER A CASUAL 31 hours of labour, we had our beautiful daughter. I still couldn't feel anything from the chest down, and after approximately an hour or so waiting for the placenta to come away on its own, it was time for medical intervention once again. The shield was back over my legs so I couldn't see what was happening, and Tommy was having some skin-on-skin time with our little girl. The poor little darling had a majorly swollen forehead from having it stuck in my cervix for about 14 hours, but to us, she was beautiful.

Dr E came and spoke to me. "Okay, so the placenta hasn't come away yet and it really should have. It's going to need to be a manual removal and given that I have much larger hands and arms than the consultant, I'm going to get her to do it." Urrgh. Her again. I appreciated that Dr E didn't want his giant limbs causing me more pain, but I didn't want this stupid woman anywhere near me again.

Thank God for the shield blocking my sight of her, and the glorious epidural that meant I didn't feel a thing. A manual removal is rather unpleasant. The consultant had her entire arm, elbow deep, inside me, using her hand to scrape away at the inside of my uterus, pulling the placenta off the wall of it. I could see my belly moving with every single scrape. Cute. Real cute.

After this glamorous part was over, my mother was wrapping our daughter up as she was quite exhausted from her birthing ordeal. Tommy was back by my side talking to me, telling me what a great job I was doing.

"Oi, have a suck on the gas, man. It's so good!" I think it made Tommy feel so much better that I was able to talk to him, and have a bit of a sense of humour after such a long and traumatic birth. He had a big suck. After seeing me hanging off it for such a long time, he assumed it must have been weak. Because he'd been awake for so many hours and was obviously in no pain, it hit him hard. He had to go and sit down for a minute.

One of the midwives then asked, "Do we have a name for her?"

I looked over at Tommy, who appeared to be concentrating very hard on not dying, and I said, "Are we going with Adeline?" We had discussed a few names, but this was the top of our list for a girl. He kind of mumbled some sort of gibberish and nodded in agreement. I spelt out the name and confirmed. Our little Addie baby was perfect. She was all bundled up and fast asleep.

It was time for us to get some much-needed sleep. While Tommy was in the shower, my mother sat beside me with tears in her eyes. She had also been by our side for the last two days and she was shattered. She said in a shaky voice, "Your sisters made birthing look

POST-BIRTH LOVE BUBBLE

fucking easy compared to that. You did an unbelievable job, and you should be so damn proud of yourself. Not very many mothers who have posterior presentation end up delivering vaginally. The best part of that birth was the friggen epidural!"

I laughed and thanked her for all of her support. My mum doesn't swear very often, so you know she is very serious when she does. "Go home and get some sleep," I said. She kissed me on the forehead and went home. I didn't find this out until days later, but when she got home, she fell into a heap and cried her eyes out. Watching your child go through something like that, especially when you help so many women have the birth they want, is extremely traumatic. She needed a good cry.

The three of us were left in our birthing suite to get some rest. Addie was fast asleep beside me, and I still couldn't feel my legs so obviously I was not moving. And Tommy was asleep on his little roll-away bed beside us. This was perfect. I was interrupted a few times by people coming in to check on Addie. Tommy was out like a light!

Mid-afternoon, a midwife woke me up and said, "I'm so sorry, darling. I left you both as long as I could but we need to get you to your room so we can free up this birthing suite."

Tommy jumped out of bed to help me with whatever I needed. The nurse removed my catheter, which I didn't even feel, and then they both helped me stand on shaky legs and head to the shower. After the manual removal of my placenta, I had blood everywhere. Tommy walked me to the shower and held onto me as I washed myself. While it's gross, childbirth and everything that happens after, I take my hat off to the partners who help women through all this gross shit. I was sitting on a chair in the shower and when I stood up, I'd left blood on it. Can't be helped given the circumstances, but Tommy just washed it off as if it was nothing.

I finally had some sensation back in my legs, so I was able to get myself changed and wheel Addie around to our private room down the corridor. I kept looking at her, not believing she was real. She was so tiny! She was born weighing a delicate 2.665kg, and 47cm long. The next 24 hours were spent in hospital, with constant observation and paediatricians coming through to check Addie's hip placement and standard reflexes. After being persistent breech for three months, she was at risk of having hip dysplasia, so I was given a referral for an ultrasound of her hips at six weeks. Everything seemed to be moving fine and there was no clicking, but given the fact she was a female and may one day have children herself, extra precautions were taken. The bruising on her forehead was honestly horrendous. She also had two perfect lines of bruising down each cheek from where the forceps had clamped on. I look back at photos of her in her newborn days and I get so teary. The poor little darling had such a hard time coming into this world, and at the time I didn't realise how severe her bruising was because I was just in a bubble of love for her.

After 24 hours we were discharged. I hadn't yet gotten the hang of breastfeeding and had cracked nipples, so we decided to stay at Mum's place for about a week until I could do it. My mother is also one of the more experienced lactation consultants in our area, so I was in the best hands. Sometimes when you have a traumatic birth, or when drugs are distributed through your body, it can disrupt the process of hormonal messages your brain sends to your body, and can delay your milk coming in. I had hardly any milk, and given the level of bruising Addie had, she now had severe jaundice. This meant she needed to be fed every three hours on the dot in an attempt to flush out the jaundice. I couldn't keep up! I ended up having to borrow breast milk from a friend, and more from some of Mum's private clients. Thank God for women and their endless flow of milk because without it, my little angel would have been in trouble.

Jen, my original midwife, came to do a home visit at Mum's house and based on Addie's level of jaundice, she advised that we needed to go back to the hospital. Unfortunately, due to the risk of exposure of infections to other newborns, I wasn't allowed to take Addie straight to maternity and instead had to go through ED (the emergency department). I was not impressed to be sitting in a waiting room with my two-day-old baby and a bunch of sick people. I made this known, and thankfully, I was whisked away to a separate waiting area.

Now, I understand the nurses and doctors in ED are exposed to all sorts of things, but if you don't know how to deal with a newborn, then find someone who does. One of the nurses was absolutely beautiful and was ever so gentle with Addie, who was extremely sleepy (this is caused by jaundice), so I didn't really mind what she was doing. One of the doctors then came in to check her temperature and was so rough with her that I honestly nearly bopped her on the head. My baby was screaming in discomfort just from having a thermometer under her arm, because this dickhead had no idea how to be gentle with a baby. After she left the room, I burst into tears. I know that I had hormones flying about, but fuck me. Have some bedside manner!

After finally being cleared to take the bili blanket home (a pad used for phototherapy to help fight jaundice), we went back to Mum's house and set up Addie's co-sleeper with the equipment. It was a bit sad seeing our tiny little baby on a blue light for three or four days. Unless she was feeding or bathing, she had to be always on the blanket. Finally, we got the all-clear with her jaundice. I had the hang of breastfeeding, even though I still didn't have enough milk and was continuously having to top her up with borrowed breastmilk; so we decided it was time to take our baby back to our own home.

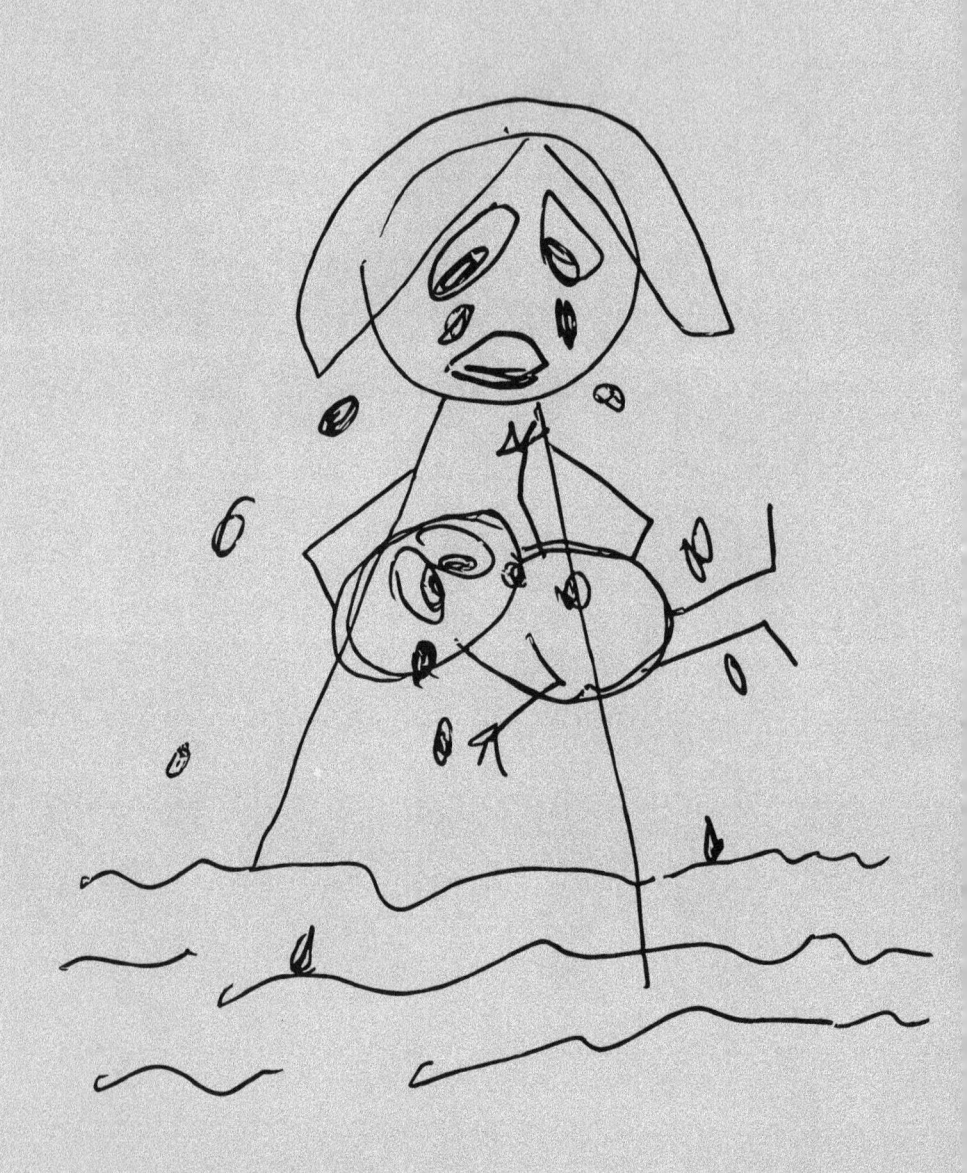

THE STRUGGLE WAS REAL

I'M NOT GOING to go into too much detail here about being a first-time mum. It's hard. Period. Every single parent goes through extremely tough times, and unless you have experienced something remotely similar on their own parenting journey, you really can't relate.

Less than two weeks post-partum, still with hardly any milk supply, I was admitted back to hospital as I had temperatures and severe pain in my lower left abdomen. I had an infection. I had a bizarre red rash on the outside of my body covering the majority of the lower left side of my pelvis, and I was shivering. On top of that, I had a sore boob with a red flush underneath it. Yep, mastitis; another infection. I needed antibiotics. I spent most of the day in hospital with a drip putting antibiotics into me. Given I also had mastitis, we did a double whammy and I took oral antibiotics for that as well. The consultant who did the manual removal of my placenta was back, and refused to believe that I could possibly have retained placenta, even though I had hardly any milk supply and an infection. Instead, I was diagnosed with having some sort of inflammation in my endometrium. Whatever. Give me the antibiotics and let me get out of here.

Most doctors will tell you that taking antibiotics is completely safe whilst breastfeeding and it will not affect the baby. I agree that it is "safe"; however, the not affecting the baby part is absolute utter bullshit. The day after I started antibiotics, my daughter turned into an absolute demon. She was screaming and writhing in agony because of what the antibiotics did to her poor underdeveloped gut. I feel so sorry for any mother who is breastfeeding and must take antibiotics. It's harrowing. I couldn't not feed her, and I couldn't not take the antibiotics for my own health, so we just had to ride out having a baby that constantly screamed unless she was asleep. And even that was tough. She rarely slept on her own, which is fair enough given she was only two weeks old, but co-sleeping wasn't working for us. She was such a hot little human, and I am also a very hot person who overheats easily; so she would push away from me and scream because she was hot, and then scream even louder because once she had pushed away from me, she no longer felt secure. It was a nightmare.

Fast forward another fortnight, after clearing her system of the antibiotics. I still had hardly any milk; I was using more and more milk from some of Mum's clients. Prior to giving birth, I had a fantastic supply of colostrum, so what was going on with my breastmilk? Mum ended up contacting Dr E, who thankfully respected my mother's professional opinion and agreed to send me off for another scan to see if I still had retained placenta. If there is any part of the placenta left behind, it can make your brain think you are still pregnant, which stops the brain from releasing the lactating hormone to bring your breastmilk through. The day of the scan came, and I had a lovely young girl who I had never dealt with before. After doing an internal scan, (yeah... three weeks after giving birth – fun) she stated, "Okay, so there is still product I can see. It's only about 6mm, but it looks like it still has its own blood supply. You're going to need a curette to have it removed." Fucking sweet.

At four weeks old, Addie was accompanying me to hospital in preparation for another procedure to have the remaining 6mm of placenta, that was telling my brain I was still pregnant, removed. I gave Addie a quick feed before I was wheeled off to surgery. Thankfully, Dr E was the one doing it for me. I only felt safe with him anyway. When I woke up after surgery, I was in excruciating pain. I needed to be on my side. The left side of my lower abdomen was nearly taking my breath away. The nurses were asking on a scale of one to ten where the pain was.

"It's a 9. Honestly, it's a 9. Please, can you give me something?"

The nurses continued to administer Fentanyl until I came down to a 7. I was wheeled back into the admissions area still in terrible pain, but I just wanted to go home and put a heat pack on it. You're not allowed to put heat packs on after surgery whilst in hospital due to the risk of bleeding; only ice. And it wasn't doing anything for my pain. I knew I needed heat.

After having a little vomit from all the medication then being able to hold down a biscuit, I was free to go. I left high as a kite. I'd been pumped full of fentanyl and Endone, so I felt very wobbly and not with it at all. I was able to feed Addie when I got home and then I had to go to bed, as standing felt unsafe; as did holding her. Two days later, my milk came in. Hooray! I was finally able to feed my daughter on my own and express enough extra to make sure she was topped up and well fed. By about five weeks post-partum, I no longer needed to borrow anyone else's milk. I was thrilled.

Addie had started showing signs of reflux maybe around the 2-3-week mark. It was hard to know for sure, I had taken a course of antibiotics that upset her gut, but her vomiting and discomfort were becoming worse. My normal GP was away so I had to see some random lady who treated me like a fragile first-time mum and told me to just put formula in my breastmilk to thicken it. Huh? Sometimes doctors need a good slap. I understand that you may deal with people who are a bit over-protective or indeed fragile. But my daughter was not well. She was in pain. Her eyes were swollen from the pain, and she only ever screamed. Why were all the other babies her age starting to smile around now, and happily lying on their backs with no discomfort at all? My baby for damn sure wouldn't do that. I left feeling upset and stupid. We had been using infant Gaviscon for a few weeks, so we continued to use that as it seemed to help her a little bit.

Christmas came and went in the blink of an eye that year. I dressed Addie up in a sweet little Christmas outfit and my family came to spend it out on the farm with Tommy's family as well. Addie had her six-week immunisations the day before, so she was a little off but nothing more than usual. Trying to be brave, we decided to go camping for New Year's, with Tommy's parents and some friends. This was a major fail. Addie's reflux hit such a severe point while we were away, and I got mastitis (for the third time by this point) again. So I was extremely sick and desperately trying to express and take

Nurofen to avoid more antibiotics, and we were stuck in the caravan with a screaming baby. Fun. Thankfully, our friends could empathise with us greatly, as their second daughter had suffered severe reflux as well, so it was great to have someone who genuinely understood what we were going through.

The drive home was a nightmare. Tommy was extremely hungover after staying up all night holding Addie so I could get some much-needed sleep, and I had to drive the car listening to Addie scream bloody murder for about two hours straight. I sat in the driver's seat with tears streaming down my face. I fucking hated motherhood. This was not how it was supposed to feel.

By the time I got home, I knew I needed help. Tommy was back at work, and I couldn't cope with this baby on my own anymore. I packed up and headed to Mum's house. Thankfully, my eldest sister was on holidays, so she came to help as well. She had dealt with reflux with her first son, so my family was well equipped to handle Addie when she was at her worst. I booked another doctor's appointment to see Dr D, who was back from her break, and I begged her for medication. She was more than happy to give it to me, as she trusted that I wouldn't have made the decision lightly. It took about three days of constantly holding Addie upright before the medication finally kicked in. My mother, Tommy, my two sisters and I took turns in shifts to keep her upright overnight, and if it wasn't my turn, whoever was on shift would wake me to feed her through the night. There were days where it would take three people to change a nappy or bath her, because she was screaming and writhing in such pain, it was impossible to do it on your own. It takes a tribe, I'm telling you!

I was in such a dark place by this point. Addie was about two months old and I was hating being a mother. I loved her, and I had this overwhelming and intense need to keep her alive; but I was so pissed off that I had been through so much and yet still had such extreme hurdles to overcome with her. It felt more than unfair. I had cut nearly all foods from my diet and was living off plain chicken, avocado, potato, lamb and rice. These were the few bland foods that wouldn't cause Addie to have major screaming episodes of pain. She was still a very unhappy baby, but it had improved slightly by this point. She was sleeping in a sitting position strapped to a chair overnight, but during the day she would only sleep on someone. I can clearly remember sitting in my mum's house one day, while she was basically jumping up and down with Addie in front of the air conditioner as it was the only way to stop her screaming and also to keep her cool, and I just hung my head in my hands. I was done. I had nothing left to give. It wasn't meant to be this tough; and it was about to get tougher.

When Addie was 13 weeks old, after I'd had mastitis for the 8th time, my milk supply was completely destroyed and I had no choice but to put her on formula. This was a very upsetting moment for me. I had battled so hard to be a breastfeeding mum. I was still expressing after every single feed right up to 13 weeks; if Addie slept for more than six hours, I would get up at 11pm every night and quietly express so that my minimal supply remained. I was using a supply line down beside my nipple into Addie's mouth and syringing extra milk into her whilst she fed from me, because I knew she still wasn't getting enough from me. I was also taking 16 tablets of Domperidone a day. Domperidone is used to help increase a mother's milk supply. I was devastated.

I trialled Addie on a goat's milk formula, and absolutely hated feeding her with a bottle. I felt useless. It felt like she didn't need me anymore and just needed anybody with a bottle. In no way did I or do I have any judgement on bottle-feeding mothers – you do what you've got to do to keep your little one happy and healthy. I just despised the fact I couldn't breastfeed. It had been taken away from me, and I was pissed the fuck off about it. I had fought so damn hard and still couldn't friggen do it. It was bullshit. Luckily, the goat's milk formula seemed to be soft enough on Addie's stomach and food sensitivities that she didn't have a reaction to it. Thank God!

From here I feel like things started to improve. I stopped breastfeeding and tried to enjoy my daughter. I was seeing a therapist regularly, trying to deal with my hatred of motherhood, which I now recognise as postnatal depression. I know that during this time everyone just wanted to help; but I just wanted to be left alone with my screaming baby. I knew I had to survive, so my relationships around me suffered. I shut everyone out and went on autopilot. Being a mother is tough, and it is especially tough when you have obstacles thrown at you before having a successful pregnancy, issues throughout your pregnancy, a traumatic birth, retained placenta, difficulties breastfeeding, mastitis eight times in 13 weeks, and a baby with severe reflux. I'm not saying my journey was harder than the next person's; what I am saying is that it was hard for me, and I refuse to downplay those first five months of my daughter's life. I know that plenty of people have it worse off. That doesn't mean that what I went through wasn't difficult for me, and that's okay.

After seeing my therapist for quite a few sessions, I felt my anger and hatred were circumstantial. Because everything seemed to be getting better with Addie, I was starting to come out of the dark cloud that I'd been stuck in. When Addie was about four and a half months old, I took drastic measures and chose to sleep train her. This was mainly because she was still sleeping in a swing, which she was now too big for, and I couldn't safely strap her in. I was worried that she would wriggle her way out of it and fall during the night. In fact, she almost did this one night, so I needed to take action.

Sleep training her was the best thing I ever did, for both our sakes. Putting her into a strict routine turned her into this contented little baby who was happy to just be. By about six months of age, she was finally the baby I had yearned for, and quite frankly deserved. Happy, well slept, content and starting to show her cheeky little personality. Finally, I knew what it meant when mothers would say, "I love being a stay-at-home mum." I did too. She was our entire world, and absolutely lit up whenever she saw Tommy, which just filled my heart. It had been a hard battle, but we made it. And I wouldn't change it for the world.

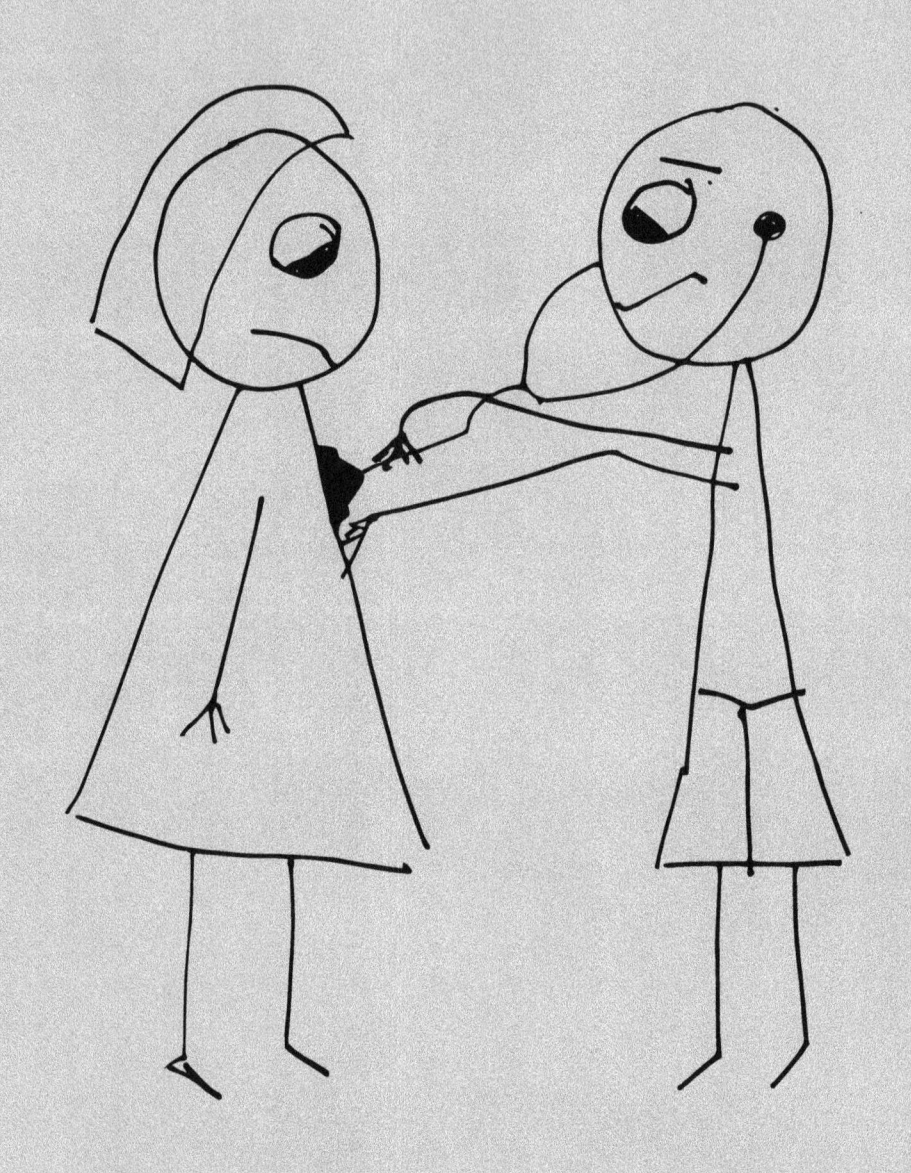

PART 3
SOMETHING IS WRONG

HAVING STOPPED BREASTFEEDING Addie in March 2019, I expected my period to return at some point. Five months later, when I still had no indication that I was going to get a period, I knew something was wrong. Most women have their period return four to six weeks after they cease breastfeeding. As you've probably worked out by now, I am far from what "most women" and "normal" are. I mentioned to my mother that I still hadn't had a period and she recommended I see my doctor. Before I did this, I opted to try taking the Pill for a month, to see if that kick-started anything. A month went by, I finished taking the Pill, and no period. Not even pain. Hmm... I still had medication from the last time my period disappeared. It was within date, so I thought I'd give that a whirl too. Religiously, for five days I took one tablet twice daily. Exactly the same as I had last time. The five days passed and still no period. Yeah, this isn't good.

I made an appointment with Dr D (my GP) and explained my dilemma to her. I was not yet ready to fall pregnant again, but I wanted to know where I was in my cycle so that should we decide we wanted to try again, we would know when I was fertile. Dr D seemed to brush off the fact that it had been five months since I ceased breastfeeding and still had no period. It wasn't until I explained that I had tried two different medications and still had no period, that she opted for a scan to see if anything showed on ultrasound. I thanked her, took my referral, and booked an appointment to see my favourite sonographer.

I attended my appointment not really knowing what to expect. The doppler was put inside me as it's a much better view. Nothing out of the ordinary. I had a thin endometrium, which confirmed I wouldn't be getting a period any time soon; but I had ovulated recently, so that was a good thing. The pictures were sent to the head sonographer for the area, and I was sent on my merry way. I went to see Dr D after the scan, to see what the report had said.

"So, the report recommends you have a saline sonohysterogram, as the possibility of *Asherman's Syndrome* could not be excluded," she told me.

Asherman's? I was convinced I had this prior to falling pregnant with Addie, and Dr D had told me it was not possible. A saline sonohysterogram (SIS) is where they shoot saline solution into your uterus to see if it is clear, or if there is scar tissue throughout. I knew something wasn't right, but the fact that I potentially had Asherman's Syndrome when I had already brought this to my doctors' attention nearly two years ago made me feel uneasy.

I had my referral for the SIS and booked in for the next available time slot, which happened to be the following Tuesday. I had never met the woman performing the procedure. I had seen her name on nearly all my scan reports over the years as she was the head sonographer for the area, but I had never met her in person. Her name was Amanda* and she seemed like my kind of woman. She was direct, to the point and kind of awkward. I liked her already. She explained to me that she would have a quick look with the doppler via internal scan first, and then perform the procedure. No worries. I was so used to these internal scans that I really didn't need the explanation, but I guess they have to do this. She put the doppler in and my uterus appeared on the screen.

"Ahh. Yeah. You've got Asherman's. Look – the other day your endometrium was like a thin pencil and now it looks like a string of pearls with all of this scar tissue." Fuck me. Of course, I had a super rare condition. "There's no point in me doing the SIS. I mean I can do it, but it's going to cause you pain and I'm not going to enjoy doing it. It's more of a diagnostic tool, but in this case, I can confidently diagnose your Asherman's without doing the SIS."

I left the appointment feeling satisfied that I had an answer but scared at the potential outcome. This meant the possibility of having any more children could potentially be slim to none. I was devastated.

I went home, where Mum was looking after Addie for me. I walked in the door and said, "Didn't need the SIS. She could see with the scan – I've got Asherman's."

Mum looked dumbfounded. She has been a midwife for 30 years and in that time she had never heard of the condition. That meant that it was indeed quite rare, or that those who had the condition weren't having more babies once diagnosed. I went back to my GP and requested for a referral be sent to Dr E so I could have a hysteroscopy and have the adhesions removed. I only wanted him to perform the procedure as I trusted him so much, and I couldn't imagine going to anyone else. I had done my research on Asherman's already and I had joined a group for Asherman's sufferers on Facebook. I felt well equipped to deal with whatever I had to do in order to sort it out.

Everything happened relatively quickly from here. Dr E saw me, booked me in for surgery at the beginning of August 2019, and put me on oestrogen for 30 days to help build the lining of my endometrium back up. I was to take oestrogen for 30 days and then for the last 10 days also take progesterone. Once I ceased taking both medications, it was expected I would have a withdrawal bleed after the procedure. The procedure itself is relatively straightforward. A tiny camera and microscopic scissors are inserted into the vagina through the cervix and into the uterus. The scissors are used to release the scar tissue. Once the procedure is complete, a catheter is inserted into your uterus with approximately 2ml of water, to keep it open. This is in an effort to stop the walls sticking back together and more scar tissue forming. The catheter stays in your uterus for 10 days. Not real glam, but hey, it's a means to an end.

During the appointment where I was booked in for surgery, Dr E dropped one of the most devastating blows I think I've ever heard. "You know I've put in my resignation, and I finish mid-September." WHAT. I was shattered. I could not go through another pregnancy without this man. He saved my life every single time I needed saving, and the thought of having to deal with someone else made me feel physically sick.

The day of the procedure came, and I was happy to see Dr E as I went in for surgery. I was very relaxed because I knew I was in great hands. When I woke up post-surgery, I again was in excruciating pain on my lower left abdomen. For about two hours I was curled over on my hands and knees while the staff were administering pain medication. When I wasn't allowed a heat pack, I lied about my pain levels and was discharged with Endone. I went straight home, took my Endone and had two heat packs straight on my abdomen. Much better. According to Tommy, I was whimpering in pain in my sleep that night.

The following morning, I woke up feeling much better. I was still a bit unsteady after the general anaesthetic and slightly tender from the procedure, but otherwise I was fine. The catheter that was still inside me had tubes coming out of my vagina and taped over to the side on my pelvis. It felt super gross every time I went to the toilet, almost like a big gloop was about to fall out; but it was just the dangling cords. So nasty, man. I was feeling hopeful that things had worked. I wanted so badly to believe that I would only need one procedure and I would be fine. Ahhhh, naivety.

The ten days passed, and I was back to see Dr E to have the catheter removed. I was ready to have it out. When he was taking it out, I didn't feel a thing; and after removing it and examining the look of my cervix, Dr E said that everything looked great.

"Thank you!" I said, as though he was complimenting my outfit. I have come to realise that after the numerous scans and poking and prodding over the years, I am so desensitised to having people up inside my bits that I have kind of a backwards set-up here. For example, I can't even look my husband in the eye during sex, but whilst a male doctor has my vagina in a forced open gape as he's examining my cervix, I can quite happily look him in the eye and discuss how it looks. Bizarre, I know.

Finally, the end of my medication came, and I desperately waited for my period to arrive. Usually within about 10 days after ceasing medication, you will have a withdrawal bleed. The key word being "usually". Me being the unusual freaking unicorn I am, ten days came and went with absolutely no sign of a bleed in sight. At about 15 days post medication, I was booked in to see Dr E.

He welcomed me into the room and said, "Okay, so you've had your withdrawal bleed, then?"

I looked at him and said, "Oh, man. You are going to rue the day you ever agreed to look after me. No, I haven't. It's now 15 days since I stopped the medication and I've not even had period pain and I don't feel like I'm going to get it any time soon."

You could see the confusion wash over his face. He relooked at the pictures he had taken whilst inside of me performing the procedure, and sat in silence for a moment.

"Okay. I think I'm going to book you in for an HSG scan with Amanda. I'm still cautiously optimistic that we got it all and you will get your period, but I think we need to check," he stated. An HSG scan is a hysterosalpingography where a catheter is inserted into the uterus and a blue dye is injected through it. This allows them, via ultrasound, to see where the dye goes and whether the uterus and tubes are open and freely take fluid through them.

Dr E wrote out the referral and told me to send him an SMS when the appointment was booked. We then realised that I would not see him again before he finished his employment with the hospital. He asked me to continue keeping him in the loop with my progress. I had explained to him that I had found a doctor in Australia who specialised in Asherman Syndrome, and if the HSG came back and I needed more work done, I wanted to be referred to this particular doctor. If I couldn't have Dr E, I wanted someone who dealt with it every single day. I wasn't risking building another relationship with a doctor only to potentially end up with this specialist anyway. Dr E understood, and was happy to give his recommendation; he passed his notes onto my GP, who would be able to do the referral should we need it.

At the end of the appointment, he hugged me. This was the final straw. I stayed strong and thanked him for everything he had done for me, and everything he did for my daughter during my pregnancy, and for allowing me to have a vaginal birth. His final words were, "Thank you, Fiona; please stay in touch." I left that appointment in tears.

With everything I have been through in the last few years, I value relationships and trust when it comes to the health professionals who take care of me. There is nothing worse than feeling like you aren't being heard or taken seriously when it comes to your own body. The thought of no longer having Dr E as my obstetrician scared the living shit out of me. For weeks after this appointment, I managed to self-induce a panic attack just at the thought of being wheeled into an operating room and it being someone other than Dr E. I can't explain to you the trust and love I have for this man. It is so intense that should I ever be lucky enough to have another successful pregnancy and deliver a baby, I have every intention of flying to the hospital where he now works, so he can be my obstetrician. The hospital happens to be on the other side of the country, so it's not like it's close, but when you've had the relationship that I have had with this doctor, you'll do anything to have them be there for you again.

I have really had to work on my acceptance of this whole situation. The strange part is, it wasn't necessarily that I was infertile. I could process that because I got my miracle baby who, based on my new diagnosis, should never have made it earthside to begin with, as everything that turned my pregnancy into that a high risk one was a symptom of Asherman Syndrome. No. It was the fact that I now had to trust someone else with my body. And that is a hard pill to swallow.

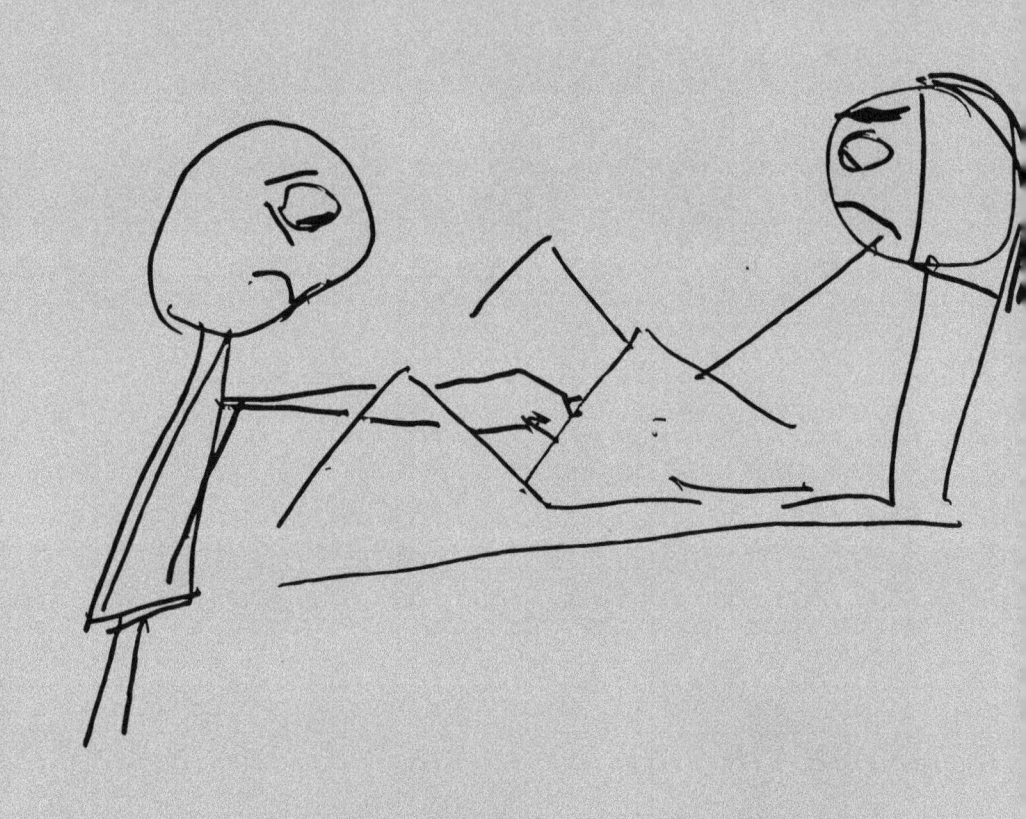

ANOTHER PROBE TO ADD TO THE LIST

WHEN I TRIED to book in for my HSG scan with Amanda, she was booked out until the beginning of October. A whole month away! I was annoyed that I had to wait so long to determine my next course of action but tried to remain positive. I had plenty to look forward to; we had a week-long holiday booked with our friends and we were so excited. It would be Addie's first big holiday. We had hired a house on an island and spent six nights there. It was amazing. It couldn't have come at a better time for me. I needed a major distraction from the stresses in my life and the opportunity to spend time with my little family and focus on the beautiful people I had in front of me; it was just what the doctor ordered.

Finally, the day of my scan arrived. I had my mother come and look after Addie while I went off for the scan. Prior to this, I had been trying to track when I ovulated so I could get some sense of where in my cycle I was. I was confident that I had ovulated the week prior to the scan and asked Amanda to check and see if this was the case, before performing the HSG. She put the probe in and was able to confirm that I had indeed ovulated recently. Great. At least I knew when I "should" get a period.

After having a brief look, she said to me, "Okay, it looks to me like the operation has worked a bit, but it still seems patchy and pretty difficult to define. We can do the HSG and see how we go; it might be pretty painful and not real fun. Or we can just leave it and I put on the report that you'll need another hysteroscopy."

Urrgh. I thought about this for a second. "No, I want to do the HSG. If I have to have another hysteroscopy, I'm going to have it done by a specialist, so I want to make sure we know what we're dealing with here."

After the decision was made, Amanda and her assistant prepped me for the procedure. This was another really glam time in my life. I had my legs up and spread, with two women crouched down shining a torch at my vagina whilst they inserted things through my cervix. For most people, this would be pretty confronting. For me, it was just another day. I didn't feel uncomfortable or awkward, and we all just chatted through it like nothing was happening. Pretty funny when you think about it. The catheter was in, and I didn't really feel a thing. In went the blue dye and we all looked to the screen to see what was happening.

"Okay, so that's fluid in the bottom part of the cavity there. But see at the top there where the fluid is kind of hitting and curling back around? That's sealed shut. So, I'm not even going to be able to get to your tubes today to see if they're clear. It's like trying to blow a balloon up that just won't work. I can't get any more fluid in there." Amanda was very matter-of-fact, which I appreciated.

"Good times!" I said. "So I'm still infertile. There's no way an egg can get through that, let alone semen get through to fertilise it, right?"

Amanda nodded. "That's correct." We finished the scan, as it was unsuccessful due to the dense adhesions sealing the top of my uterus shut.

I had not taken Amanda to be empathetic in any way; as I said, she was very blunt and to the point, which is what I liked about her. Then as she took everything out of me and took her gloves off, she rubbed my knee and said, "Sorry. I know that's not the outcome you wanted. We'll give you a minute to get changed."

A massive ball in my throat rose and threatened to explode. Why did people have to be so nice? "Oh well," I said, "it had to be some sort of outcome, so at least I know where to go from here."

She looked at me sadly and said, "You will need to have someone release that top part regardless. It's for your own health. You still have built-up blood in the back of your pelvis."

I understood. I had already found the specialist; now I just needed my referral and I could get the ball rolling. I explained my plans to Amanda. She had heard of the specialist and also added that she knew of a few women who had seen him, and went on to have successful pregnancies. This gave me hope.

I got home and managed to hold it together when I was telling Mum what had been found in the scan. I could see she was devastated for me. I contacted the specialist's office, which was in a different State, and asked to know what I needed with my referral to ensure a smooth process to become one of his patients.

"Just send through any scans or photos confirming diagnosis and he will review them; then we will contact you for a phone consultation given your location."

Great. I was booked to see my GP the following week and was ready to get this ball rolling. I was so scared. The thought of trusting someone else to perform this procedure was really beginning to stress me out. I had been through so much with different doctors performing curettes on me before finally finding Dr E, who was the most caring man I could have ever hoped for, only to be thrust into someone else's hands and expected to simply trust them. This was going to take some time for me to get my head around. I could feel a panic attack building and I needed to get it under control before I actually had to go through with it.

The following week I went back to my GP, Dr D, and went through the scan results and what I wanted to do moving forward. She was very much in agreement with me going straight to a specialist; having been an obstetrician herself, she didn't want me to have more damage caused by having different doctors poking around in there, regardless of their skillset. She did the referral while I was there, gave me a copy to send away, and faxed a copy straight to the specialist's office. Awesome. I could get this ball rolling. That afternoon, I emailed a copy of the referral, along with photos from my procedure. The following morning, I rang the office to confirm it had been received.

"Yes, we have it. It's sitting with him to review so once he has had a look, we'll probably call in a day or so to book you in for the phone consult," the office lady explained. Fantastic. I felt like this was going smoothly already.

I received a phone call the following day from another office lady, who advised she had had a cancellation and could fit me in for a phone consult that Friday. Just three days after the referral had been sent. Unreal!

"Yes, please," I said, "that'd be great."

I then booked my sister in to take Addie swimming for the Friday morning and arranged for my mother to be here to listen in on the phone call in case I missed anything. It all happened so quickly. The specialist called me and after thanking me for my very detailed referral, he went through the process.

"Surgery is to be done on Day 3 to 12 of your cycle. On Day 2 of your cycle, you will commence Progynova, which is to delay ovulation. The maximum I will have you take that for is ten days. The morning of your surgery, you will come to my office, and I will withdraw some of your blood and remove the platelets. The platelets will then be used once the surgery is complete, to assist with healing the uterus and building up the endometrium. If it is Stage 2, you will be free to try and conceive right away. It it's Stage 3 or 4, you will need to have an HSG scan first to confirm everything is open or if another procedure is required. Obviously, I won't know what stage your adhesions are until I am performing the procedure. After a successful procedure, the rate of conception is 87%. Now, that is conception only, and it does not mean you may not miscarry, okay?"

I liked this man. He didn't dick around and he got right to the point. I got a great vibe from him. Everything he said sounded perfect. We finished the phone consult and he told me I would hear from his office ladies to book the procedure in. Given that I was on Day 5 of my cycle, I knew I had about a month before it would happen. I was ecstatic. I felt great knowing that he had such a high success rate. I just wanted to get this happening.

I continued to track my ovulation from Day 5 and ovulated bang on time. This meant I knew exactly when I would get my period, so I was able to book in for surgery. I contacted the admin ladies for the specialist and was confirmed for surgery on November 13th, 2019. The day after Addie's first birthday. My scripts arrived so I could commence progynova shortly after, and we booked our flights. My mother came with us so that there was an extra person to be with me at the hospital and someone to take care of Addie as well. Everything seemed to be falling into place.

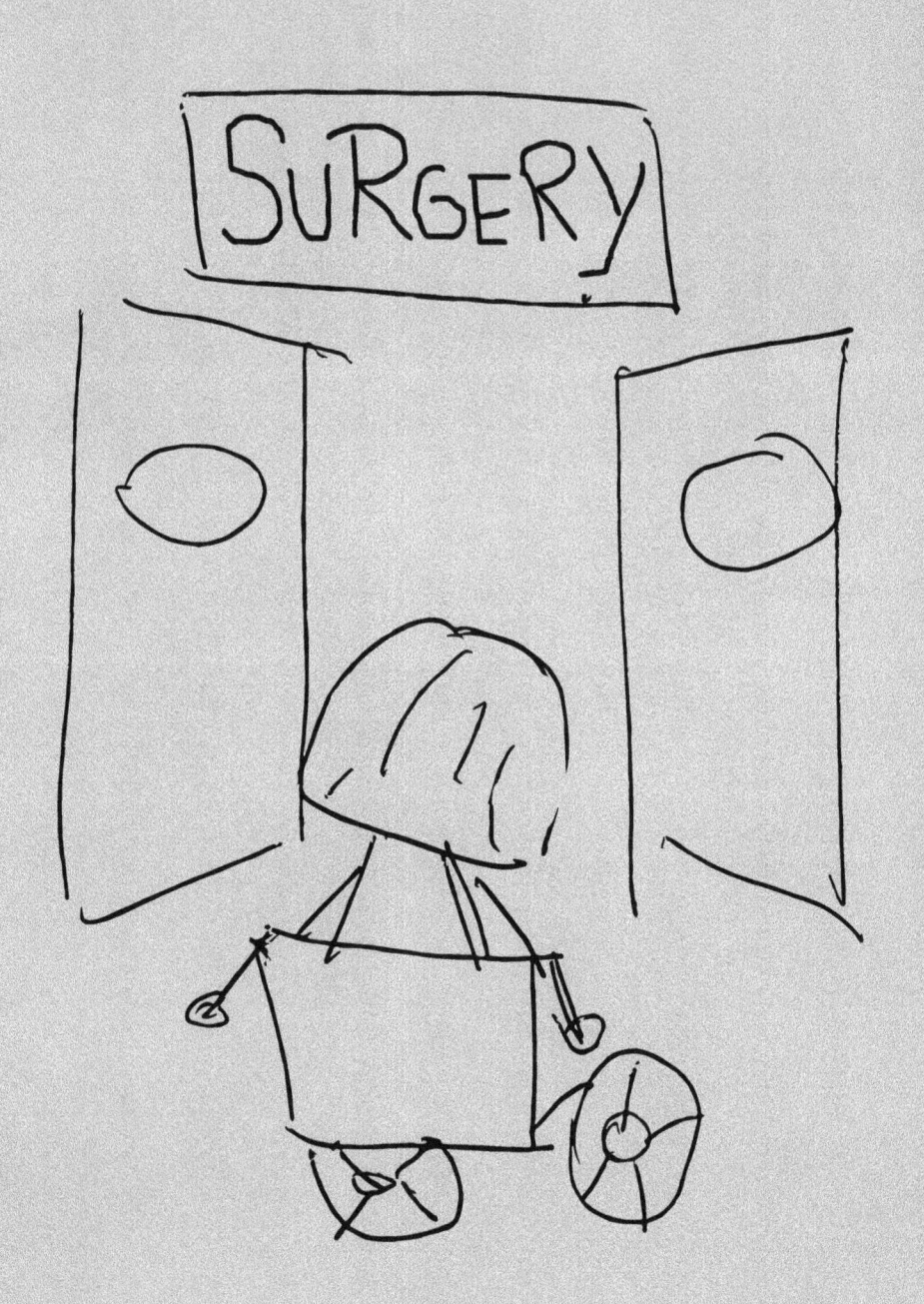

SURGERY NUMBER WHO KNOWS WHAT

THE WEEKEND BEFORE we were due to fly out, we celebrated Addie's first birthday. It was an emotional day for me, as I'm sure it is for every mother. I looked at this beautiful little girl who just lit up my life and hoped that one day I would be able to give her a sibling. I could feel the yearning in my soul for another child. Even though Addie had been far from easy, I knew I would do anything to make it happen. Of course, we dressed her in an obnoxious outfit, and she made everyone smile. She got to enjoy her first ever cupcake, which she obviously inhaled. We went with a rainbow unicorn theme; she was our rainbow baby after all, and a bit of a unicorn because of the fact that she was never meant to make it here with all the difficulty we'd had throughout my pregnancy with her. But hell, she made it! We were so damn proud of her.

Mum, Tommy, Addie and I all caught our flight on the afternoon of the 12th November 2019. Addie did well on the flight, even though she was not feeling herself and suddenly had become a bit sick. We made it to our destination late that evening and were lucky enough to be able to stay in my aunt and uncle's house while they were away. It was close to the hospital and had plenty of space for all of us. The following morning, we decided that Tommy would stay home with Addie and Mum would come with me to the hospital. Thankfully, I no longer had to go to the city first to have my blood drawn, as the specialist had notified me that he now had the ability to do all of this in theatre. It meant we could spend the morning down at the beach, getting some fresh air together before I had to head to the hospital for surgery.

The time came for me to go to the hospital. I thought I was doing well stress-wise. I said goodbye to Tommy and gave Addie a kiss, then Mum and I caught an uber to the hospital. I sat in the front of the car as I tend to get motion sickness, and as we pulled up to the hospital, I nearly lost my shit completely. I could feel panic rising in my throat, and I wanted to get out of the car and run. What the hell was I doing? Why was I trusting someone I had never met in person to essentially clean my insides out? I felt sick.

"Get your shit together, Fiona," I said to myself quietly. "Everything will be fine. Just breathe." I closed my eyes and breathed deeply for the last part of the car ride. Who'd have thought Calmbirth breathing techniques would be so helpful in the most random of situations!

We found our way to the relevant ward, and I had to sign some paperwork as I was checked in for surgery.

"I nearly had a panic attack as we were driving in here," I said to Mum. "Just the thought of someone new and having to just trust them is really scary. I know he is at the top of his field, but it doesn't make it any less scary."

Mum looked at me with sadness in her eyes. As a mother myself, I know you want to take it all away from your kids and take on the pain or fear yourself. I often forget what I have put my poor mother through. Lucky she is tough! It was nice to be able to spend some one-on-one time with Mum. Even though the circumstances were a bit ordinary, it's not often we get to spend so much time together. I was so glad she was there with me. Not that I didn't want Tommy at the hospital with me – I would have been happy with either one. But at that point in time, I think Tommy needed some Addie time in his life rather than hanging around a hospital all day.

Finally, my name was called to go into surgery. Mum gave me a hug and wished me luck. As I was wheeled away from her, I could feel myself start to panic. Holy shit, this was happening. Breathe, girlfriend. I still hadn't even met the specialist. Was I going to? Or was I just going to be put to sleep and never see the man? I was placed in another waiting room just before the theatre and met my anaesthetist. He was a lovely older man, and I think he could tell I was a bit wound up.

I tried my best to act calm, and I think I did a pretty good job; but he put my cannula in and said, "I'm just going to give you some Valium to relax, okay?" As soon as I felt the Valium rushing through my body, I was so thankful for it.

Suddenly a man covered head to toe in PPE and with a mask covering his face popped up and introduced himself as the specialist. "I'm just going to draw your blood, Fiona, and we'll separate the platelets to put back into your uterus after surgery. It will be wonderful for your healing. You okay? See you in there."

He was a man of few words, and I was high on Valium so I couldn't have cared less about what he was about to do. I fell asleep before I was wheeled into theatre. It was glorious.

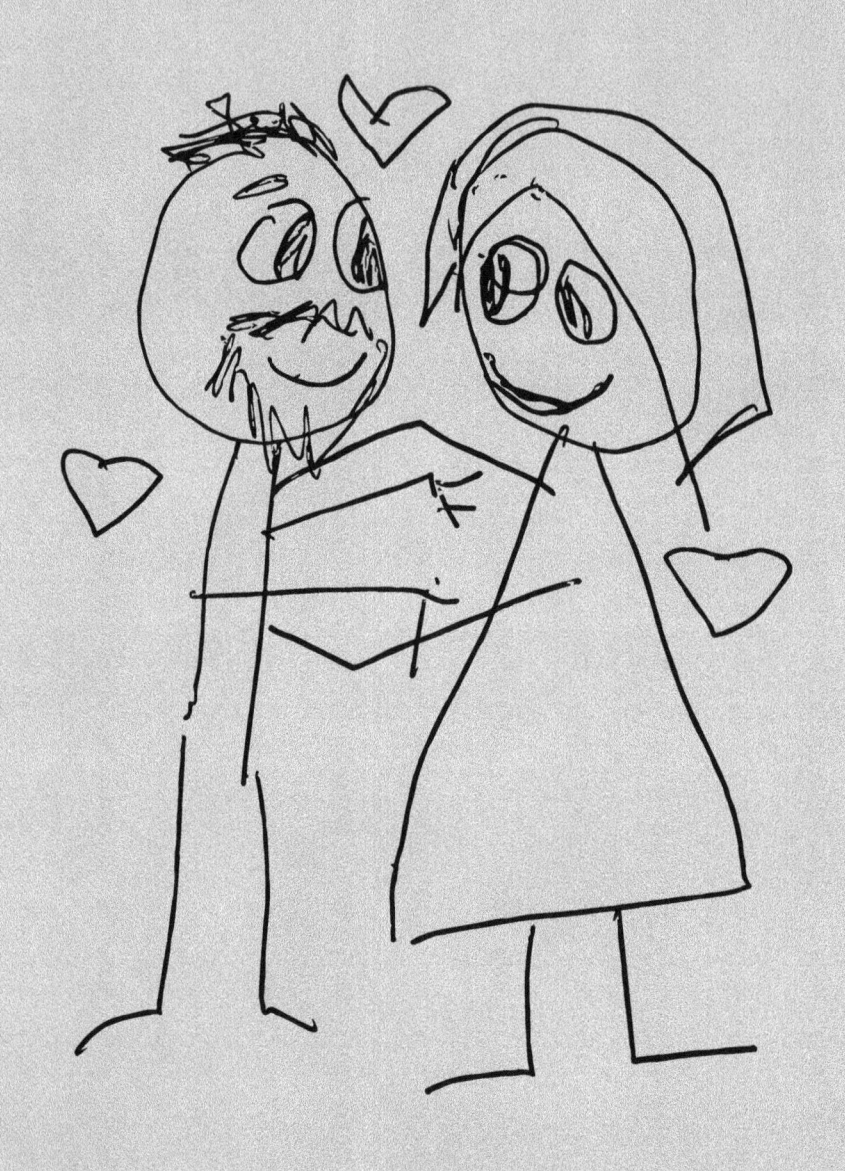

WE GET THE GREEN LIGHT

I WOKE UP in recovery and surprisingly felt no pain whatsoever, but man I felt sick. I wanted to vomit. I answered the pain questions and went back to sleep. Given that I was still high as a kite, I had no idea how long I had been in recovery. I do remember them telling me my blood pressure was super low and they wouldn't let me out of recovery until it had returned to what it was pre-surgery. I always had low blood pressure after surgery, so it wasn't anything new to me. I finally got wheeled into the waiting room, still feeling sick as a dog, and handed food that I obviously had to eat before I could be discharged.

Mum came flying into the room with big wide eyes, going, "Are you all right? What took so long in recovery?" Poor woman. Being a midwife, she obviously knew roughly how long recovery would be, but apparently I had been in there significantly longer and she had got herself so worked up as to why.

"Yeah, I'm fine. I'm not in any pain at all. I just feel queasy. My blood pressure was low; they wouldn't let me out of recovery until it got back up to what it was before the operation. Why? How long was I in recovery for?"

Now, my family has a tendency to be a tad dramatic. "Oh my god, I thought they'd forgotten about you, and you had brain damage or something!" Mum was frantic. I burst out laughing at her. It wasn't funny for her in the moment, but seriously who would suddenly think that brain damage was the reason for the longer time in recovery?

I was able to eat the food handed to me – an egg sandwich. I felt much better after eating it. I just had to be able to pass urine before I was allowed home. I kept drinking water to try and make it happen, but it was taking forever. I started to feel sick again and as I was walking to the toilet to try and wee, I knew I needed to throw up. Yep, up it all came. An egg sandwich in reverse is one of the rankest things I've ever thrown up. Yuck! After another 40 minutes when I still hadn't been able to pass urine, I decided to lie and say I had. I was sure it would be fine, I just wanted to get home to my baby for a cuddle. It was after 6pm by the time I got home. Addie was tired and emotional and just wanted me. I was still woozy but happy to be home with her.

We all had an early night that night, and finally at about 11.30pm I was able to pass urine. Phew! It's the strangest feeling sitting on the toilet trying to wee and having absolutely nothing happen. My bladder was obviously woozy from being put under.

I recovered well from the surgery – minimal bleeding and hardly any pain. I was just tired. We spent two more days there and then parted ways in Melbourne. Mum was going to visit her mother, and we were headed to Bright for Tommy to compete in the Spartan Ultra Marathon that weekend.

I received an email outcome from the specialist about my surgery. It was short and sweet, and answered all my questions:

> *Hi Fiona, surgery went well. You have stage 3 Asherman Syndrome, the scar tissue was successfully removed and PRP instilled. Please continue antibiotics for up to 7 days and progynova for another 10 days. The treatment is considered complete, so you can attempt conception at your leisure. If you're not pregnant by the end of April 2020, please contact us again. Let me know if you want me to give you a call for further discussion or questions. Regards*

Geez. I wasn't expecting to be given a timeframe for conception! From what I understood the PRP (platelet rich plasma) therapy lasted approximately three months, so if I wasn't pregnant by the end of April 2020, I would potentially need more surgery as the risk of scar tissue returning was quite high, plus I would need to have more PRP. My head was spinning. I was thrilled that I didn't need another scan to check everything though. Now, it was just a waiting game as to when my period would return. In the meantime, it was time to enjoy our family holiday in Bright and Melbourne.

Seeing Tommy compete in the Spartan Ultra was one of the proudest moments of my life. He rang me at the halfway mark to let me know how he was going and gave me a rough time for when he would be at the finish line, so that Addie and I could cheer him on. For some reason, I felt he wasn't giving himself enough credit, so I decided to be there 40 minutes before the time he gave me. As I was walking into the Spartan area towards the finish line, my phone started ringing with Tommy's name across the screen.

"No! We didn't miss you finish?" I said as I answered the phone.

"I'm done, babe. Where are you?"

I couldn't believe it. I was devastated that I'd missed seeing him on the home run. Having been a competitive athlete for nine years of my adolescence, I knew how amazing that final rush was when you're hearing people cheer your name, and I was really upset that I hadn't been there with Addie cheering him on for his final steps.

When Addie and I made it to the finish line, Tommy was smacking a beer and certainly didn't look like he'd just run 50km and completed however many obstacles! We worked out that if he had registered for his age group, he would have received a silver medal. He completed the Ultra in 9 hours and 28 minutes. As I said, it was one of the proudest moments of my life.

When I first met Tommy, he was a typical 21-year-old party boy who would do anything to get on the piss with the lads; and at times he could be painfully selfish in doing so. Here he was five years later, still a party boy at heart, but dedicated beyond belief to improving his fitness, mental health, and all-round bettering himself as a human being, and I was bursting with pride. He had come a long way from the young man I had met five years earlier, and seeing him so happy and proud of himself is a memory I will cherish forever.

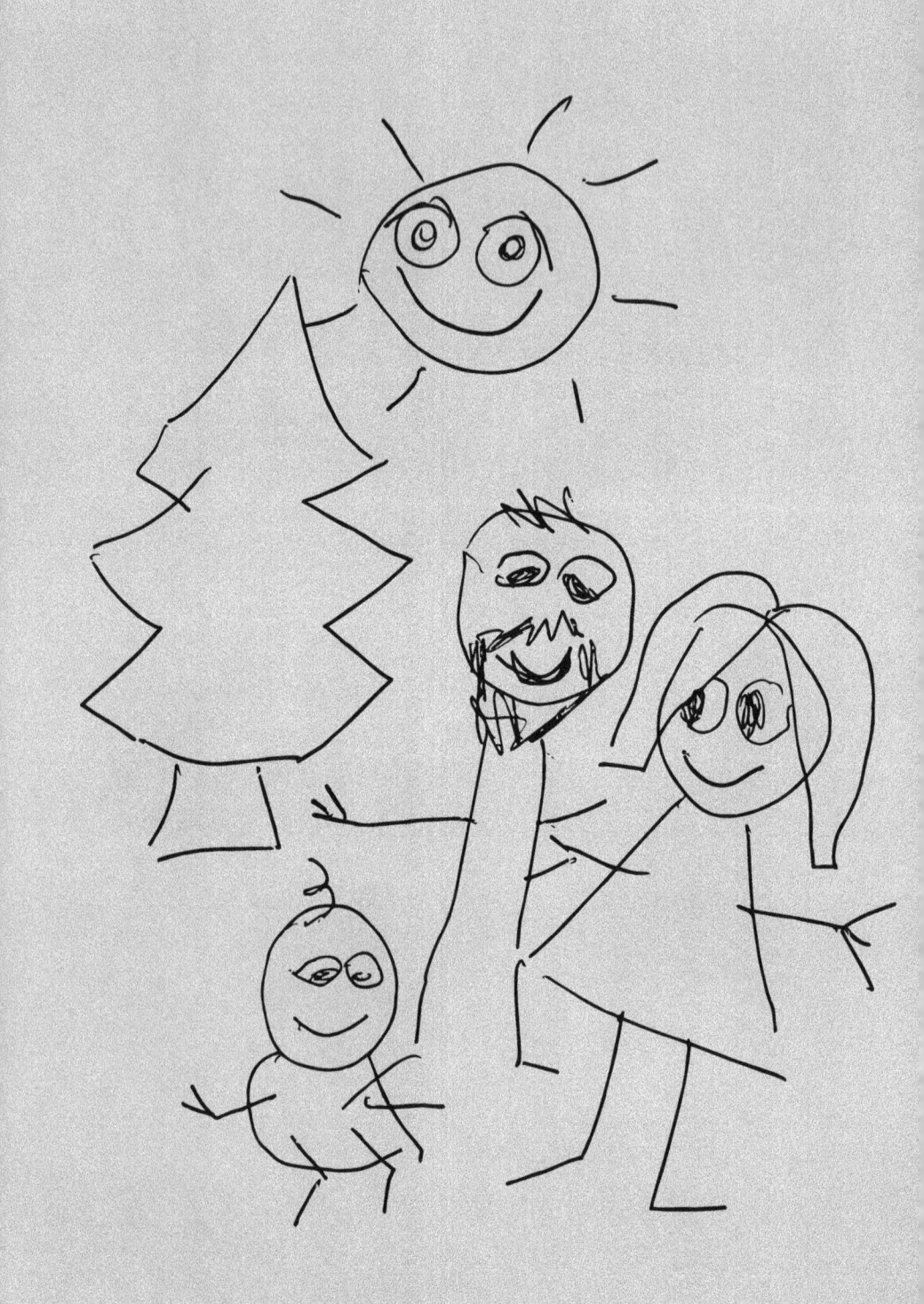

LIFE GOES ON

OUR HOLIDAY CONTINUED, and after Spartan we spent some time with my grandmother, which was lovely. The cool weather was perfect, and it's not very often I get to see my Nana, so spending a few days with her was wonderful. Addie just adored her, and Nana loved having Addie around. It was a special time for all. I left Tommy in Melbourne as he had a work conference to attend, and I flew home with Addie by myself. Two flights later we were home, safe and sound.

I had done some research on Asherman Syndrome and joined a support group on Facebook, and I started to gather information on what I could potentially do to reduce the risk of scar tissue returning. In one of our phone consults prior to surgery, I had asked the specialist if there was anything I could do. He had bluntly advised no, but then indicated that acupuncture might help. From my own research, I found that inflammation was a leading cause of scar tissue forming. So I started looking into an anti-inflammatory diet and identified that gluten and dairy were some of the leading causes of inflammation in the body. I am by no means a dietician, nor do I have any medical or educational background myself to support any of this information. This is simply what I have gathered from my own research.

The Saturday I returned home from Melbourne, I decided to give up gluten, dairy and sugar cold turkey. I left Addie with my mother and decided to go grocery shopping. I bought my last caramel cappuccino and enjoyed it in peace while I bought food to support my new way of life. Addie was already dairy and gluten free, so I mostly ate this way anyway. However, I still had dairy with my morning coffee and the hidden gluten and milk solids in nearly EVERYTHING, so I was cutting it all out. For the first three days, I was very angry and irritable. Everything everyone did annoyed the absolute piss out of me. I remember thinking, *When did everyone get so goddamn annoying?* – only to realise I was the problem. Funny, that. After about a week I started to feel a lot better. I booked in to see my acupuncturist and started having regular acupuncture with him to help reduce inflammation in my body, and hopefully keep the scar tissue at bay.

On December 5th 2019, I had what would be considered a "withdrawal" bleed. I had ceased the Progynova the fortnight before and finally had bright red blood, something I had not seen for an extremely long time. I considered this to be Day 1 of my cycle, but as Christmas was fast approaching, I decided against tracking my ovulation and figured if I was meant to fall pregnant this month I would. I just wanted to make sure I had a "normal" month and that my cycle had properly returned.

That year we spent Christmas with my family. Copious amounts of alcohol were consumed, as well as plenty of gluten- and dairy-free treats for me. I was thrilled that I had made it over a month being gluten- and dairy-free, and I was feeling great for it. I was starting to get severe reactions from foods that had the warning "may contain traces of gluten". I would blow up like a balloon and look about six months pregnant just from things that "may" contain it. I started to see how bad it really was and had no interest in reverting back to eating it. I was due to get my period on January 2nd 2020, based on my standard 29-day cycle. Leading up to it, I started to feel all the right ways – moody, fragile, irritated, and just generally a headcase. The date came and went, and a few more days passed, and I got no period. What the hell? I didn't get any pain either, so I knew I didn't actually get a "period", but I had no idea what was going on.

The following week, I returned to work after 14 months off, which I thought I was fine with. At the same time, Tommy had to be out of town for three weeks, so I was by myself getting Addie off to daycare, dealing with the hormones of a period, and returning to work. I ended up taking five days of Primolut in the hope of making my period start, because I felt like a nutcase. I needed a hormone reset and I needed it bad! I took five days of the tablet and still no period. To say I lost my shit is an understatement. I booked myself in with my GP and demanded a saline (SIS) scan with Amanda again. Thankfully, she had a free spot for January 21st 2019, so I snatched up that appointment as quickly as I could.

Tommy returned home from work, and I unleashed. Poor guy. I know now that I was clearly not coping with returning to work. I felt he had no idea about what I was going through and by simply saying, "You'll be right, babe, you'll find your groove with it," he was belittling my feelings or just brushing them off. I felt unsupported. In hindsight, I was a hormonal crazy bitch who was being a tad dramatic. But at the time I was a raging bull. I can remember sitting on the couch with Tommy, trying my hardest to have a rational conversation about how I was feeling, and suddenly screaming at the top of my lungs, "I don't care if you think I'm some sort of crazy bitch, Tommy; I'm trying to tell you I'm not okay and you're not fucking listening to me!" He burst out laughing at me. He actually laughed at me. Not the best reaction, bud, but I can see his point. I rarely had outbursts like that, and to him, it was obviously funny because it was so unexpected. Laughing at someone in the midst of a meltdown, though – not helpful. I threw more expletives at him, and stormed off crying out of pure frustration and fury at him.

Ahhh, men and women. We are such different creatures. After I had calmed down, we sorted everything out and had a good laugh at what a psycho I had just been. One of the greatest things I love about our relationship is that we can find the humour in the shittiest of situations and the biggest of arguments. If you can't laugh at yourself then you're taking life way too seriously. Life is already hard enough without being able to find humour in the strangest of situations.

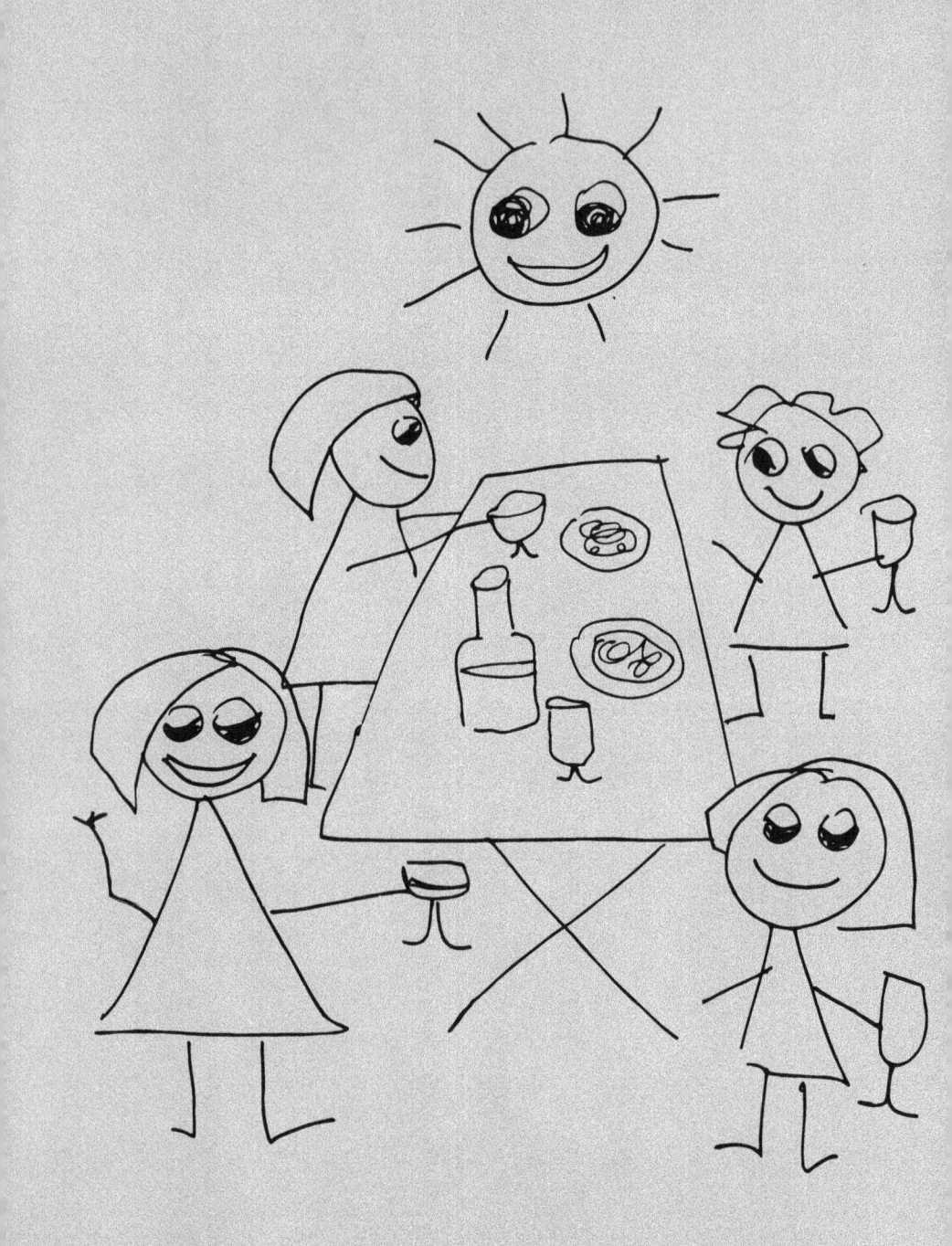

SOME GOOD NEWS AT LAST

MY SCAN WITH Amanda rolled around and Tommy was able to come with me. Not that I needed him for moral support, but more because I wanted him to meet Amanda and he was available, so why not.

"Hello again," I said to Amanda as we walked into the same scan room, as I always did.

"You brought company this time? What, are you scared of what I'll do to you?" she asked jokingly.

"Not at all! Tommy was just available so figured he could come and see what's going on too."

Basically, we were going to be checking that everything was clear. Amanda explained to me that we would put a catheter into my cervix, and she would shoot saline into my uterus to see that the uterine cavity was clear and that fluid was able to flow through my tubes as well.

Once again, I had two women shining a torch at my vagina and inserting what they needed to in order to get the job done.

"You're not going back to work after this, are you?" Amanda asked me.

"Yeah. I'll just take a Naprogesic afterwards; it'll be fine," I said.

"Jesus. You should be having the rest of the day off!"

We continued with the procedure and watched the screen to see where the fluid went.

"Okay," Amanda said, "everything looks really good. Your uterus is clear, and the fluid is free flowing. The patency of your tubes looks great too, so I'd say the surgery was a success. He is great at what he does, that man!" I felt a flood of relief. "Looks like you're coming up to ovulation as well. Probably in a week or so." Oh, thank God. Hopefully, if I could track my ovulation, I would know exactly when I was meant to get my period. Amanda finished the procedure and removed the catheter. "Whatever you do, don't stand up – it's a mess down here!"

I laughed and said, "Yeah I can feel it."

I cleaned myself up and when Amanda returned to the room, she reconfirmed her findings. I was very happy with the results and now just had to track my ovulation in the hope of knowing when a period was due.

I thanked Amanda as I left and she said to me, "How about next time I see you, we work on having something to actually look at?"

I burst out laughing and said, "Look, I'm working on it, all right!" I really liked her. She was odd, blunt, and awkwardly funny. My kind of gal.

I tracked my ovulation and got a positive ovulation test, so I knew I was due for my period 14 days later. Having returned to work, I had filled the girls in on where I was at in my life with all of this, and they were all now deeply invested.

On February 10th 2020, I woke up to go to work and went to the toilet. When I wiped, I had bright red blood. HOORAY! Bang on schedule, my period had arrived. I was so excited. I decided to wear a pad, which I never do usually, because I wanted to see how much I was bleeding. Sounds rank I guess, but unless you've experienced no bleeding and longed for your period like I have, you probably wouldn't be able to understand.

I sent a text to my mother in my excitement, saying something along the lines of, "Is it weird that every time I go to the toilet and wipe I kinda wanna frame how much blood I'm getting?" Again, I know this sounds rank.

Mum totally understood my excitement and I received a text message back saying, "DO IT!!"

Like I said, unless you've been in this situation you probably can't understand how exciting it is to feel normal again. I went to work and proudly told the girls I had gotten my period. They were so excited for me that we all decided to go out to lunch to celebrate. Period party! Any excuse for a lunch date, really. However, this was pretty exciting.

Tommy and I decided to track my ovulation once again and just see what happened. I didn't want to put too much pressure on falling pregnant, as I didn't want to become obsessed with it as I had prior to Addie. When we put pressure on ourselves, I felt like it just ended in miscarriage, and I didn't want that to happen this time. The plan was to track my ovulation and if we were in the mood then we would have sex, but if Tommy was out of town or we were too tired or life got in the way, then it wasn't meant to be. I can't remember exactly what happened that month – from memory, I think Tommy went away for work the day I got a positive ovulation test so in my head we had probably missed it. We had had sex a few days earlier, so part of me was hopeful; but at the same time, I wasn't holding my breath.

I was due to get my period on 10th March 2020. Four days before that, while Addie was having her daytime nap, I was sitting on the couch eating lunch and something suddenly told me to take a pregnancy test. At the time I thought it was stupid, but I couldn't let it go. So I said to myself out loud, "This is going to be negative; you should just wait a few more days." Anyway, I took the test and left it on the bathroom counter. I cleaned up my lunch while I waited and went back into the bathroom to have a look. There it was. Two lines on the test. The second line was faint, but it was definitely there. What? We did it? Oh my god! Tommy wasn't home and wasn't due home until late that night. I decided to keep it to myself and retest the following morning to see if the line was clearer.

The next morning, I got up early before Tommy and took another test. Positive. This time the line was ever so slightly darker. Jesus! I decided to surprise him. We've never been able to do a cute surprise or get excited about a pregnancy, so I thought why not treat this one a little bit differently. I got Addie up and we had breakfast together. I placed the pregnancy test in an egg carton and after Tommy got up and had a coffee, he sat down to play with Addie.

I gave Addie the egg carton and said, "Ta for Daddy." She took it and handed it to him happily.

"Oh, thank you!" said Tommy and put it down.

"No, open it," I said. He opened the egg carton and picked up the test. He looked at me and said, "Are you pregnant?" I smiled and nodded. He was so happy! He leapt up and gave me a big hug. "We did it! That's awesome, babe. Thanks for that surprise too, what a nice way to find out." We were so happy to finally be able to be excited about a pregnancy.

I waited until after the due date for my period had passed to let Mum know I was pregnant. A few more days went by and by Friday 13th March 2020, I knew something was wrong. I sat in Mum's house and said, "I'm not pregnant. It's gone, I'm sure of it." She tried to tell me to be positive, but in my soul I knew. All my symptoms had disappeared, and I just knew it was gone. Tommy had a buck's party to go to that night, so even though he offered to stay with me, I bid him farewell and told him to have fun.

The following morning, I was so anxious to know what was going on that I got a blood test form from Mum and went to check what my blood levels were doing. In my heart I knew it was gone, but my anxiety had gone into overdrive thinking about my next move – how I was going to get it out. I didn't want another curette as that is what had potentially caused so many of my problems with Asherman Syndrome and infertility, and I didn't want scarring to come back tenfold.

The only options I had were to have it come out naturally, which could take months if it was a missed miscarriage, or to have misoprostol again, like I did with the twins. I just needed to know what was happening so I could decide on a direction. Once again, Mum told me to be positive and it was most likely just my anxiety playing tricks on me. I went and got the bloods, but I wasn't too interested in the results as I already knew the answer. By about mid-morning, just after I got home, I started bleeding. I knew my body and I knew it well. I messaged Mum to let her know I had started bleeding and she replied with my blood results. My HCG was 4. The pregnancy was gone.

I had a baby shower to attend that afternoon, so I put Addie down for her nap, threw myself in the shower, had a big cry and dusted myself off. I did my hair and make-up and put on a new outfit – fake it to make it, right? It turns out that going to the baby shower was probably one of the best things I could have done. I was able to focus on someone else's happiness and run around after Addie, who was having the time of her life. I didn't bleed a lot with this miscarriage; less than my period the month before. But I was so worried I had retained product and would need to take the medication anyway.

A week after I had stopped bleeding, I arranged a referral for a scan to check for retained product. I was terrified. I just didn't want to have to deal with this shit again. I walked into the scan room and the sonographer was a young girl who I had previously had scans with, and I think she recognised me. She was satisfied that no retained product seemed to be visible, but a report would be completed by Amanda and sent to my doctor. Seeing the report, I could finally relax. No retained product was visible, and my endometrium lining was measuring a thin 2mm. By this point, it was mid-March and given that I really did not want to have a Christmas baby, and also had no idea what my cycle was going to do, Tommy and I figured we had missed the boat and would be back to see the specialist in April for further surgery. Great.

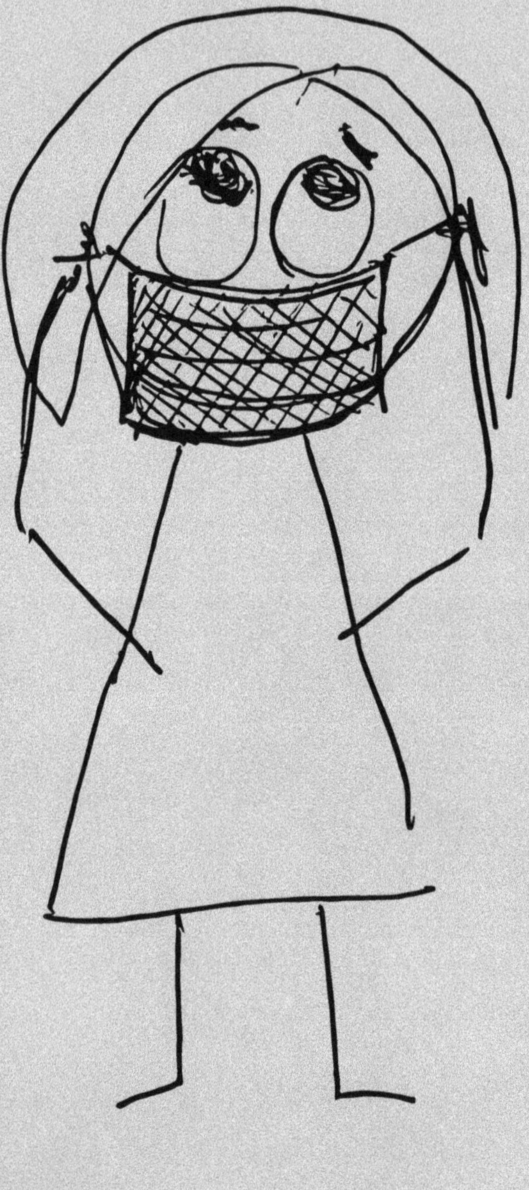

PART 4
THE PANDEMIC

IT WAS AROUND this time that Australia went into full-blown lockdown. It was a scary time for everyone, and I was already so terrified of losing Addie, that I completely shut everyone out; I social distanced hard. I did not want to put her at unnecessary risk. Looking back now, it was a tad extreme, as regional towns in our State were significantly safer than other places. However, at the time it was all fresh and frightening for everyone.

As the world shut down, all elective surgeries, including infertility/fertility treatments, were put on hold, and I assumed I wouldn't be having surgery in April. I didn't know what my cycle was going to do either. I had read on the Asherman's support group page that several women suggested taking a high dose L-arginine supplement, which was extremely effective in thickening the endometrium for successful implantation. L-arginine is essentially a protein builder, and my understanding is that for successful implantation of an embryo, the lining needs to be a minimum of around 7mm or more.

Keep in mind, at my scan a week after my miscarriage, my endometrium was measuring at a measly 2mm. I figured I had nothing to lose in trying out this supplement so I ordered it and commenced the recommended dosage these women suggested.

It was quite a large dose - 6000mg per day. Each tablet was 1000mg, so it was suggested to take three tablets in the morning and three at night, then once you got a positive pregnancy test, slowly wean off by one tablet per day for a week. For example, five tablets a day for a week, then reduce to four per day for a week, and so on. Usually by around the 12–13-week mark of pregnancy, you should no longer need to take it. My plan in taking it, even though I didn't want to become pregnant right away, was more to give my endometrium time to thicken.

About two weeks after our miscarriage, Tommy brought home some drinks for me to try. I was particularly enjoying ciders at this point, and he thought I might like a cider mixed with champagne. To say it was pure rocket fuel was an understatement - it was something crazy like 2.4 standard drinks per bottle! I remember drinking the first two while Tommy was drinking Great Northern mid strength (so one standard drink per bottle) and he was trying to make me keep up with him, drink for drink. Apparently, I got two more in, and I can vividly remember saying, "Dude I am off my head." That's the last thing I remember. When I woke up the next morning, boy, was I sick. Tommy wasn't even the slightest bit dusty, and I asked him if we had had sex the night before. He gave me a very detailed run down of my performance which, given the state I can imagine I was in, sounded extreme. I looked at my phone and realised it had been two weeks exactly since our miscarriage, and thought I should probably do an ovulation test just to see where I was at. After throwing up, I took an ovulation test and crawled back into bed.

I got back up a few hours later (Tommy was on Dad duty) and felt slightly better. I went to check the ovulation test and staring back at me was a smiley face. Shit. I was ovulating and we had unprotected sex last night.

I walked out to the kitchen and said, "So I just got a positive ovulation test and we had sex last night!" Tommy just stared at me. "If I fall pregnant it's going to be due, like, Christmas Day!" I said, sounding horrified.

"Would that be such a bad thing?" he asked.

Something in my gut was telling me this would happen. I really did not want to have a Christmas baby, but at the same time, I wanted another baby. I went back to lie down and continue trying not to die from the rocket fuel.

Five days after I got the positive ovulation test, Tommy and I had sex. I went to the toilet afterwards, and I looked at the toilet paper after I wiped – a habit I continue to have whether I am pregnant or not and for some reason am always waiting for blood. I had to do a double take because it was pink. I was spotting. This never happened after sex. I didn't mention anything to Tommy and went to bed. The next morning, I had this overwhelming feeling that it had been an implantation bleed. It seemed ridiculously early to be having it, but my gut was telling me that was what was happening.

I said to Tommy, "So I think I'm going to be pregnant this month and I think it's going to stick. This is it. I'll bet my life on it." He believed me – I was so in tune with my body and after explaining to him that I had had some spotting the night before, he also felt the same way.

Tommy went away for work the following day and was out of town for a few nights. Eight days after I ovulated, I was playing with Addie after we'd had dinner, and once again got an overwhelming feeling to go and take a pregnancy test. I tried to talk myself out of it because eight days post ovulation meant I still had six or seven days before my period was due, and the likelihood of the test being positive was extremely low. I didn't want to feel disappointment.

Of course, I did a test anyway. Ever so faintly that second line appeared. It was faint, but dammit, it was there! I still have a photo of it on my phone and I can still see the faint line.

Tommy rang me that night shortly after I had done the test, and asked me how I was feeling. "You've taken a pregnancy test, haven't you?" He knew me way too well.

"Yeah, I have… and there is a faint line," I said.

We turned the phone to Facetime and he could see it too. It was still a week before my period was even due, and the line was so faint anything could happen. But something kept telling me I was going to stay pregnant.

I waited until I was due for my period, which was 12th April 2020, and took another test that morning. The second line appeared so quickly and it was extremely dark and thick – darker than the control line even! I was so happy. This was it; we were having another baby and it was going to be due on Christmas Day.

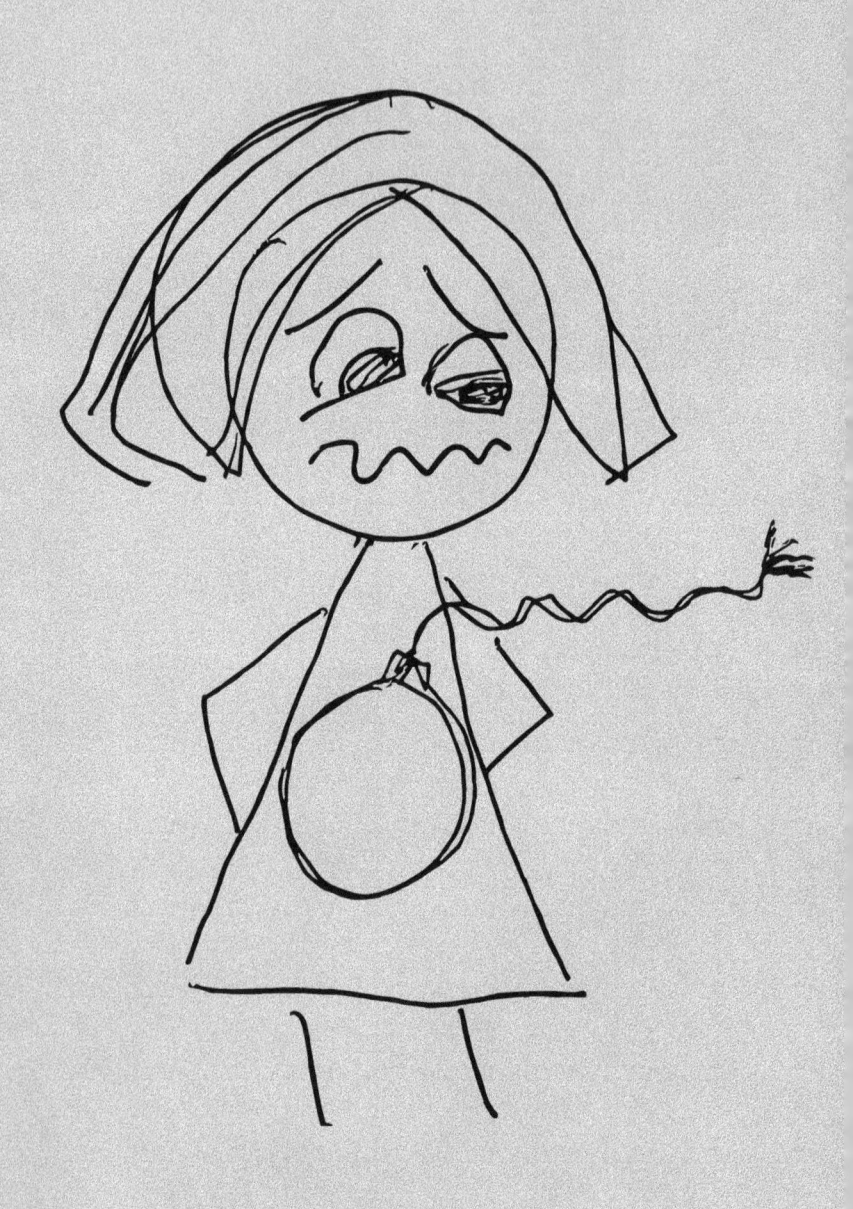

PREGNANCY AFTER LOSS

AT AROUND THE six-week mark, I woke up feeling queasy and threw up. Fantastic. Even though I was so sick through my pregnancy with Addie, I loved throwing up every day because it was a constant reminder that the baby was still there. At six weeks and three days we got a scan of our little bean, and there was a heartbeat. It was measuring perfectly, with an expected due date of 22nd December 2020. I was so happy. A few days later, though, all the sickness disappeared and I convinced myself I had lost the baby. It was gone, I was sure. My wonderful mother arranged another scan for me as I was so sure it was a missed miscarriage. My boobs still felt sore, but I was no longer feeling at all sick, and had even convinced myself I wasn't tired. Tommy was devastated. He kept asking me, "Are you sure?" And I kept saying yes, I was sure.

I went to the scan alone as by this point, Covid rules restricted the number of people who were allowed in the room. I walked into the familiar room with a sonographer I had never met before, and quietly waited for her to start. She put the doppler inside me and I waited for those four dreaded words: *There is no heartbeat.* I stared at the roof, mentally planning my next moves and what I would do after this appointment.

"There we are, beautiful little heartbeat flickering away there. See?" she said, turning the screen to me.

"Are you fucking kidding me?!" I blurted out and started crying. "What a little toad! All my symptoms are gone so I thought for sure it was gone!"

She laughed at my reaction, and I felt a wave of relief wash over me. I have never left one of these appointments ringing or texting people saying I still had the baby. Never! This was my 6th pregnancy, so I had left these early scans four times previously after hearing those four words that utterly break your heart. Instead, some sort of miracle had happened, and my baby was still alive.

I skipped out of the appointment, raced to the car and sat there for a minute, crying. I rang Tommy and sobbed down the phone, "We still have a heartbeat!"

"WHAT? Are you SERIOUS?" He was just as shocked as I was, and so damn thrilled. "I was not expecting that at all, babe. that's amazing!"

I texted my mother as well, and she was so happy for us. Surely my anxiety would now be laid to rest, and I could focus on enjoying this pregnancy.

Of course, this was not the case. Pregnancy after any kind of loss is terrifying. With Addie I had been lucky that I threw up every single day until about 18 weeks, by which point I was able to feel her moving so my anxiety was eased. This time around, having been sick and then having the sickness vanish, I felt more confused and anxious that something was wrong. I managed to make it through another fortnight, by which point I begged for another scan just to make sure the baby was still there. At nine weeks, the baby still had a super strong heartbeat and was developing perfectly. I made a deal with myself to try and make it longer than a fortnight before having another freak-out that the baby was gone.

At around the 10-week mark, I was sitting on the couch and I could swear I was feeling movement. It was low, and ever so subtle, and if I wasn't so hypervigilantly aware of any and all sensations in my lower abdomen, then I probably wouldn't have even noticed it. It definitely wasn't gas; it was the unmistakable flutter of early movements of my baby. It was almost as if the baby knew I needed reassurance some other way and was making it known that everything was okay in there. At 11 weeks exactly, I decided to ask Mum to try and get the heartbeat on the doppler. This is super early to try and do – we had managed to get Addie's heartbeat on the doppler at 11+5, so I was hopeful this time would be the same. Mum put the doppler low on my belly and aimed downwards towards my toes. As loud as anything, a beautiful heartbeat could be heard!

I had said to Mum that if we were able to get a heartbeat on the doppler, then I was happy to share with the family the news that I was pregnant. I was starting to show already, and it was getting harder to hide. At my birthday dinner that week, Tommy and I shared our exciting news. Everyone was thrilled. My eldest sister had a much better reaction to this pregnancy than she did to Addie's, and all our nieces and nephews were excited to be having another baby to add to the family.

For some reason, something kept niggling away at me throughout this pregnancy. I knew I didn't want a Christmas baby, and something told me I wouldn't have one. In my head I kept trying to convince myself that I would go overdue by about 10 days and would have the baby in 2021. At around the 17 weeks mark, I went to the toilet and when I wiped, there was thick gloopy brown discharge on my toilet paper. Fuck. Given that it was brown, I was confident that perhaps it was just old blood and it had mixed with standard discharge. I rang my mum, and she immediately came over to check the baby's heart rate. Bub was still happy heartrate-wise; I could feel it moving and didn't get a sense that anything was wrong. I contacted Dr E, who was more than happy to hear from me, and put my mind at ease about the discharge being brown. He assured me that he felt confident it would disappear within a few days. Thankfully, he was right. Once again, he came to my rescue when I needed it.

The weeks rolled on and for some reason I just couldn't bring myself to publicly announce that I was pregnant. With Covid restrictions still in full swing, I was working from home so no one really saw me, which meant I was able to keep this pregnancy to myself. We obviously told our family and close friends, but I couldn't shake the feeling that I didn't want to announce it in case something happened. I put it down to the fact that I had lost so many babies that I was just going to have to deal with this anxiety the whole way through. The anatomy scan rolled around and at 21 weeks everything looked great. My cervix was long and closed, bub was developing perfectly, and at this point it didn't appear that I had any issues with my placenta. The cord insertion was great, there was a few extra parts to my placenta but nothing to be concerned with. As each week passed, a sense of relief came with it.

It was around this time that I started feeling extreme pressure in my vagina. It honestly felt as though it had puffed up and was about to explode! Naturally, I grabbed a mirror to see if that indeed was the case, but it all looked normal. There were no obvious signs of veins being exposed or swelling in any way. But it felt as if I had varicose veins and almost as if they had their own heartbeat. Thankfully, we were still working from home at this point, so I was able to sit with an icepack on my vagina for most of the day, which was very helpful in relieving the pain and pressure. As I have said before, pregnancy is just so glam. Here I was with what felt like swollen flaps and an icepack in my underwear, whilst dealing with customers complaining about electricity loss. Just living my best life.

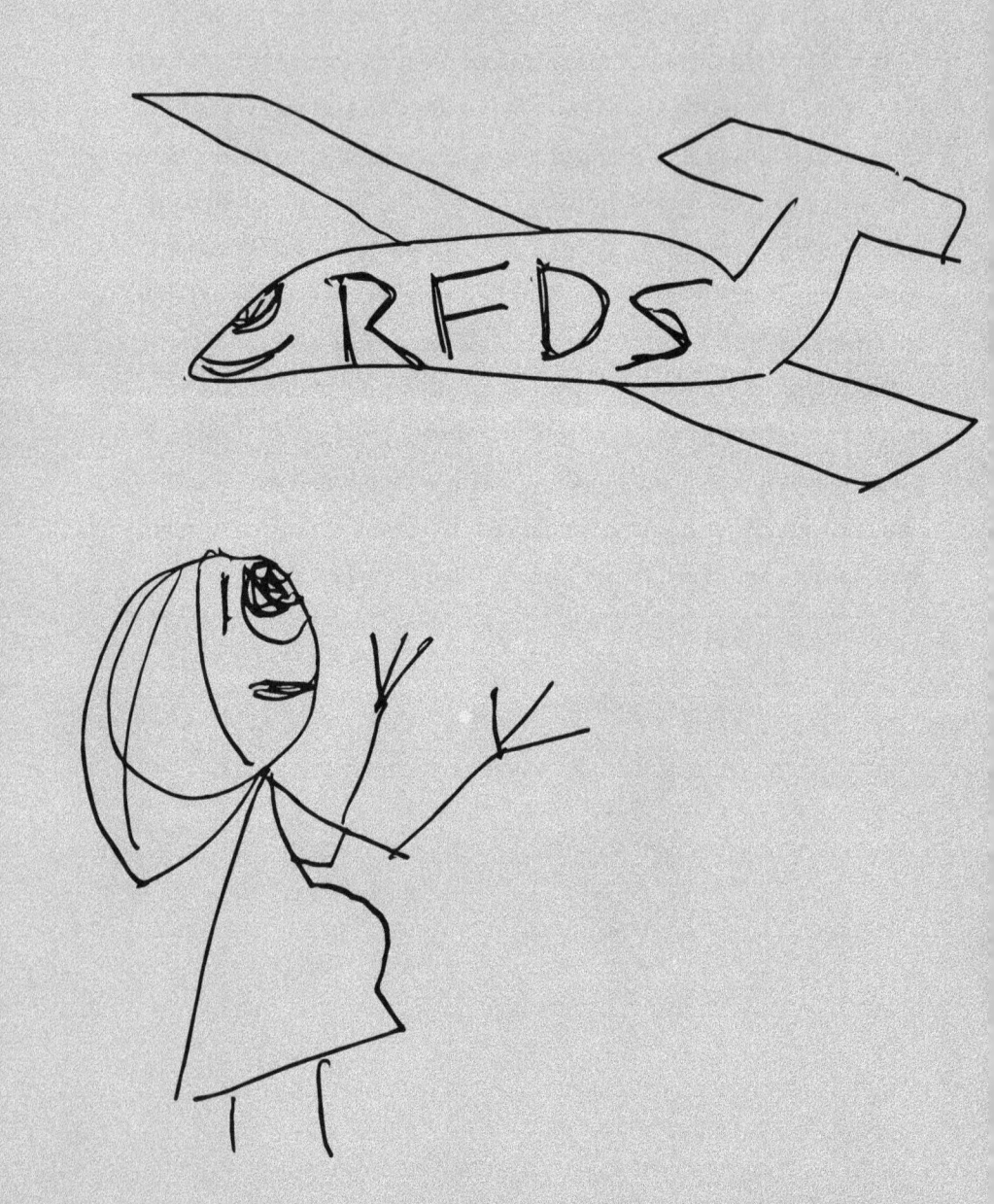

WHEN THINGS GO WRONG, THEY GO REALLY WRONG

AUGUST 31, 2020. A night I will never forget. At 23 weeks and 6 days gestation, I sat down in the bathroom so I could play with Addie while she bathed. As I sat down, it felt like a big gloopy blob fell out of my vagina. Now, for anyone who has been pregnant, discharge is a given. I assumed this is what it was and thought I would clean it up right away before helping Addie bath. I went to the toilet, wiped, and instinctively looked at the white paper. In my hand was bright red watery blood, along with what appeared to be my mucous plug. Holy shit. I immediately told myself to breathe. I could feel the baby kicking, and my gut was telling me that the baby was fine but I needed to get checked out ASAP.

I called my mum, who was busy at the time. I contacted my midwife and sent a photo of the bloody toilet paper. She rang me straight back and we agreed to meet at the hospital at 7 pm. It was approximately 6.30pm by this point. Tommy had just walked in the door, and I said to him calmly, "I've just had some bright red bleeding so I'm going up to the hospital to get checked out. I can still feel the baby moving and my gut is telling me it's okay, so I will give you a call once I've been seen." He looked alarmed but trusted my gut feeling and wished me luck. I left without even saying goodnight to Addie, as I assumed I would see her in the morning.

I met my midwife on the ward and she took me into one of the rooms to wait for the registrar to come and do an internal. I was hooked up to a CTG and bub's heart rate was perfect. Given that my mother works at the hospital on the maternity ward, everyone knew who I was, and the registrar was quite excited to meet me. She was a young woman with dark hair and a kind face. She explained to me that she would be putting a speculum into my vagina to open it so she could get a better look at my cervix. No problem – get up in there, girl. The speculum was in, and a light was shining into my vagina. She went quiet. Then she popped her head up from between my legs with eyes as big as saucers. "I've never seen this before," she said. "Get the consultant," she directed my midwife.

I don't think my midwife actually picked up on the seriousness of the request, mainly because I gave a bit of a laugh and said, "Of course you haven't! If I had a dollar for every time a health professional said that to me..." I rolled my eyes and laid my head back down to stare at the ceiling and begin my process of dissociation.

The registrar still had her hand on the speculum, which was holding me open at this point, and again stressed to my midwife the urgency.

"The consultant is just with another patient, but I'll go down and see if I can grab her. Do you maybe want to explain to Fiona what you have seen?" my midwife said as she walked out to find the consultant.

"So, Fiona, what I think I'm looking at is your cervix partly dilated with some of the amniotic sac actually exposed through your open cervix. But I want the consultant to have a look before we do anything more."

My mind was racing. I knew what this meant. I would be flown to a Level 5 hospital as soon as possible if labour couldn't be stopped, and either the baby would die after being born so early, or I would have to give birth to an extremely premature baby who potentially could be deformed or disabled for the rest of its life. Fuck me. "Awesome," was all that I could manage to get out.

The consultant entered the room. She is one of the most beautiful and gentle women I have met. The registrar explained to her what she thought she was looking at. The consultant bent down to have a look in my vagina, nodded to the registrar, then came and stood up beside my head and said, "Okay. This is shit. Do you want us to do everything?"

I stared blankly at her and said, "Yeah, of course."

She carefully explained that they would contact the Royal Flying Doctor Service and arrange my evacuation to a larger hospital, where I would be kept close to the Neonatal Intensive Care Unit, unless of course they were unable to stop the labour, in which case the baby would be delivered that night and we would both be evacuated. Fuck me.

"Can one of you please ring Mum for me and I will ring my husband?"

The consultant left the room to call my mother. I rang Tommy and when he answered I just said, "Sooooooo, I'm being transferred to a bigger hospital tonight. They've had a look and I'm 3 cm dilated with bulging membranes. So, part of the baby's sack is actually visibly out of my cervix."

I waited for his confused response. "What the fuck?" Yeah dude, my thoughts exactly.

Tommy contacted his parents to ask them to come in and stay with Addie while she slept so he could be with me until I was evacuated. They lived about 40 minutes out of town, so our beautiful neighbours came and sat in the house until they arrived so that Tommy could leave right away.

Before Tommy arrived at the hospital, my mother appeared. I will never forget her face. She walked around the corner into the room with big wide eyes and in pure shock said, "I never expected this." It wasn't until later that I found out she had walked past the consultant who was on the phone to the Rescue Service and overheard her say, "The parents have requested full resuscitation." What a statement to hear about your unborn grandchild! At this point, she didn't know what was going on or what had been identified, as the consultant had only called her and explained she was extremely concerned and that I wanted her to be with me. I filled her in.

I don't know whether this is standard procedure for all threatened premature labour or if there is a gestational cut-off for it, but I was hooked up to a machine that pumped high doses of magnesium into me, which research has found to be extremely beneficial to the baby's brain development. It was around this time that Mum arrived, and I was trying my hardest to breathe through the genuine fear of exploding into flames with how hot I was while the magnesium was going in. This was a heat I had never experienced. My face had turned bright red like a capsicum, and I was sweating profusely. I had to get Mum to wet towels and put them on me, plus find a fan to blow cool air onto the wet towels. I was still burning up under there! Keep in mind that it was the middle of winter, so everyone else had jackets on and were even colder with the fan going, but I felt like I was in an oven.

Prior to the magnesium starting, the consultant had done a quick scan to check on baby and make sure it was far away from my cervix. Bub was frank breech, which is exactly what we wanted at this point – as far away as possible from my dilating cervix.

"Given that this is all going to shit, can you please tell me whether it's a boy or a girl?" I asked.

"Are you sure?" she said to me.

Tommy and I had been clear that we didn't want to find out the gender, but at this point, I wasn't sure if this baby was going to live or not, so I needed to put some sort of connection in place by confirming the gender and potentially deciding on a name.

She searched around and said, "It's a boy." Of course it is, I thought to myself. A little boy to absolutely terrorise me. Tommy walked in a short time later looking like he'd seen a ghost. He kissed me on the forehead, asked why I was so red and covered in wet towels, and asked if I was okay.

"I got the consultant to check – it's a little boy," I smiled. He seemed happy with the news, but the whole situation was extremely overwhelming.

In the background of all of this, the hospital was in the process of contacting the Rescue Service to arrange a Royal Flying Doctor Service (RFDS) flight. A woman had been transferred approximately 30 minutes prior to when I had presented, and by the time the plane was able to get back to collect me and then return, it wouldn't have been able to land in the fog. A decision was made to leave me until the morning. As luck would have it, one of my mum's close friends was working for the Rescue Service at the time. When she saw my name come through as requiring evacuation, she knew it would have been serious and desperately tried to help me. As the only other NICU in the State, another Level 5 hospital was contacted, and they were happy to accept me. An RFDS flight was also available. A specialised midwife was sent on the pending flight in case I gave birth mid-flight and we waited for collection. It all seemed to fall into place for us, whilst our whole world felt like it was crashing down.

While waiting to be evacuated, Tommy raced home to pack a few things for me like toiletries, a change of clothes, and a phone charger. We weren't entirely sure if Tommy would be allowed on the flight with me, so he packed a few essentials for himself as well. Mum stayed with me and told me to try and get some sleep. The lights were turned down in the room and all that could be heard was the constant blip of our baby boy's heartbeat on the CTG. Mum sat beside me while I tried to sleep, and I can remember opening my eyes at one point to look at her. She sat with her head bent down just staring at the ground, gently rubbing her hands. I could tell she was praying. As my eyes filled with tears, I closed them again and tried to pretend none of this was happening to me.

Tommy returned shortly before the evacuation team from RFDS arrived. I had been told that before I could be evacuated, a final internal needed to be done to check whether I had dilated any further. If I had, we would need to deliver. I prayed and hoped with everything I had that labour had been stopped. I knew I didn't want to have this baby here. Something in me told me I just had to keep him in a bit longer and get to this bigger hospital where we would be safe. The RFDS crew arrived in the early hours of the morning on September 1st 2020. A new registrar came in, introduced herself and explained that she would be checking to make sure I hadn't dilated further. She told me that if I had made it to 5cm we would need to deliver, as the baby was so small and being frank breech there was extreme risk of not dilating fully and the baby dying on its way out. Cool.

Once again, the speculum went in. The lights were still low in the room and yet it felt like there were so many people standing around. Tommy was up near my head and Mum was somewhere close by too. The registrar was down between my legs, my midwife was in the room, 2 RFDS officers were by the door, and the specialised midwife was also in the room. My whole body started to shake and shudder and I started crying. This terrified me. Please, I begged my body, please still be at 3cm. We are not having this baby here. No. I pushed my face into Tommy's chest and sobbed, trying to hold still for the registrar to effectively check my cervix, but also having absolutely no control over the terrified shuddering that my body was producing.

Finally, she spoke. "Still 3cm, Fiona. Labour has successfully been stopped."

Oh, thank God. I think we all breathed a sigh of relief – there was still a tiny bit of hope that this baby might make it. One hurdle down, a million and one obstacles to go.

From here everything felt surreal. I had this underlying sensation that everything was going to be fine, and by that, I mean I didn't feel like we were going to lose this baby. I held onto it as hard as I could. I was wheeled out by the RFDS team and was backed into the elevator on a bed. I was to remain horizontal at all times. I kissed Tommy goodbye, with his plan to race home and grab a few things and start the eight-hour drive to the bigger hospital. Mum gave me a big hug and she managed to hold it together enough to tell me to stay positive and keep praying. As the elevator doors closed, I waved goodbye to Tommy and Mum, tears welling up in my eyes as they turned to each other and hugged, each probably feeling as helpless and shocked as the other.

I kept thinking to myself, *Why? Why is this happening?* Sadly, it's a question I have had to ask myself so many times, and to this day, I do not have the answers.

NICU

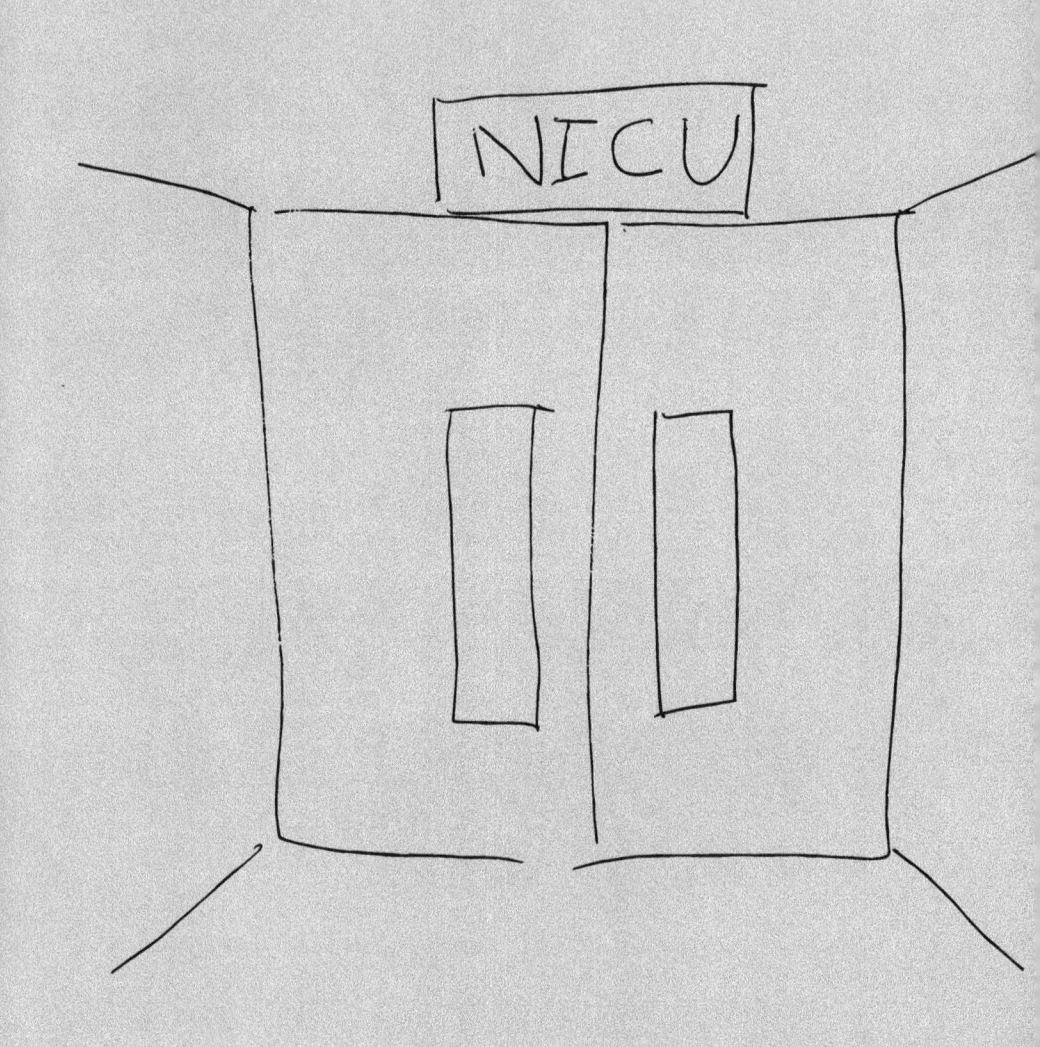

OUT OF OUR DEPTH

I WAS TAKEN via ambulance to the airport, where the RFDS jet was waiting for me. Paperwork was completed, more monitoring of myself and the baby was done before take-off, and as I watched the lights of home disappear as we took off, silent tears streamed down my face. I kept thinking of Addie and how her little brain would process that Mummy was gone. I didn't know when I would see her again and it tore me apart.

It was a relatively short flight, and aside from all the drama, I can remember thinking that flying whilst lying down was absolutely the way to go. I get horrible motion sickness, so being forced to be lying down for take-off and landing was amazing. There was a bit of a delay once we landed, as the wrong ambulance was sent to collect me. It was a nice opportunity to find out more about the RFDS officer and his background. They really are wonderful people, and his care and attention could not be faulted. I was absolutely his

Number 1 priority, like some precious cargo, and I couldn't help but think how lucky I was to have this man in charge of my transfer.

Upon reaching the Level 5 hospital, I was quickly wheeled into the birth suite for further monitoring and to discuss with the consultant what the plan was. A scan showed that my cervix had stayed at 3cm and I was no longer contracting. By this point, it was approximately 4am and I was exhausted.

"Given that you are not in active labour and your cervix has stopped dilating, I don't see the point in rushing you off to theatre," the consultant explained. "We will monitor you closely for the next few hours and as long as nothing changes, we can hopefully admit you to the ward. We will book a scan for later today with our MFM (Maternal-Fetal Medicine) and go from there. Obviously, the longer we can keep the baby in the better. Happy?" She was lovely. I love it when people are direct and get right to the point with me.

I was left in the care of a midwife, texted Tommy and my mother to give them an update, and tried my best to get some sleep. This proved very difficult with 30-minute observations needing to be performed on bub's heart rate. The midwife was so careful though, and I can remember I was too tired to even move for one of the OBS, and she just gently worked around me while I wearily nodded that it was okay for her to proceed. I was told that a scan had been booked for lunchtime, and thankfully Tommy arrived just in time to come with me. The hospital we had been transferred to hadn't been as severely impacted by Covid-19 so restrictions were not as strict, which meant I was allowed to have one person in the room with me.

From here, a lot of what I was told is a bit of a blur. I am so glad I thought to record part of my journey by doing a short video on my phone of where things were at. I hate watching it, though. It makes me cry every single time; mainly because I can feel how much pain my heart and soul were in. But in terms of reminding me of things, it is great. We started the scan with a lovely lady and then halfway through the MFM specialist, Dr F* came in to have a chat with us. He was a quietly spoken man, but I liked him right away as his bedside manner was right up my alley.

Dr F explained that my uterus clearly wasn't very receptive to a placenta, as it had tried to attach anywhere it possibly could and was basically everywhere. He showed me on the screen where parts of the placenta appeared to have died off. At the time of this scan, I was 24 weeks exactly and baby was weighing approximately 690 grams. Dr F advised this was a good size for positive outcomes for survival; around 70%. The longer I was able to keep the baby in, the better the outcomes in terms of disability or brain damage.

"Are you finished having children?" Dr F asked me.

I looked over at Tommy and then looked back at the doctor. "Uhhh, I think all of this will pull me up, so yeah." I couldn't think of anything worse than having another pregnancy at this point, when this one had gone so catastrophically wrong.

"With having Asherman's and how your placenta looks, if it doesn't come away or I can't stop the bleeding, I'm going to have to remove your uterus. It will be a full hysterectomy. I just want to make you aware of that."

Prior to getting pregnant, Tommy and I were fully aware of the outcomes in terms of my uterus if we were to be successful in holding a pregnancy. We knew that a hysterectomy would be inevitable to keep me alive if I had placenta acreta or haemorrhaged.

"Yeah, that's okay. We knew that would be a possibility before getting pregnant so that's fine," I said.

We left the scan with a picture of our tiny baby boy, and both felt we were in safe hands. I was admitted to the ward with a room of my own, and we both got some much-needed sleep for the afternoon.

The next 48 hours were long and hard. Tommy had managed to get a room at the Ronald McDonald house just across the road, which meant he was about 200 metres from the entrance of the hospital. I basically had to be on full bedrest, only getting up to go to the toilet (which was a tough experience in itself) or shower, and every time I went to the toilet, there was blood when I wiped. I was wearing a pad to catch it as well. I have always said that pregnancy is a nasty business, and I stand by that statement wholeheartedly. I can remember being so scared to poo in case I accidentally pushed my cervix open. It was a real low point when I had to hover over the toilet and hold pressure on my perineum while trying to poo, out of pure fear that this baby was going to fall out of me into the toilet! Like I said, pregnancy is a nasty freaking business.

At 24 + 1, I had a slow leak of fluid, so was whisked off to the birth suite for some monitoring and to make sure I wasn't contracting or dilating. Thankfully, neither was the case so I was allowed back onto the ward. I really liked this hospital. The staff were lovely, and the doctors were so vigilant; I felt that we had been sent to the right place, even if it was a million miles away from our little girl. We had tried to go for a tour of the Neonatal Intensive Care Unit (NICU) since we had arrived, but unfortunately it just hadn't worked out. On the afternoon of 24 + 2, we were booked in with one of the nurses so that we would have been exposed to the floor if the baby was to come. I had tried to pre-warn Tommy that it might be extremely confronting seeing these tiny babies, and that they would be all skin and bone with lots of tubes and wires. I didn't want him to feel overwhelmed. For some reason, I wasn't scared of what I was going to see.

At around 4.30 pm a wheelchair was brought to my room and Tommy wheeled me around to NICU for our tour. As soon as we entered, we met a lovely nurse who explained to us the rules of the unit. Given that the patients on this floor were extremely vulnerable, cleanliness and hygiene were of the utmost importance, and everything was to be sanitised before going any further. Hands washed, phones wiped, and accessories removed and put into a locker; we were then given the tour. We were shown babies around the same gestation as ours, and also babies who were born around the 24-week mark, and were told how they had progressed. I remember walking past rooms, and the nurses would smile, and the parents would kind of just look at you. I smiled at them, hoping they would be reassured; sometimes you got a smile back, other times it was a blank stare. I didn't think much of it at the time, but now – now I know that look.

We finished the tour and were given a small bag with gifts inside. A book on what to expect, a teeny tiny beanie for the baby, a notepad and stickers to record milestones, and other information leaflets. As we left NICU, we felt good. Our goal was to at least make it to 26 weeks, but we both agreed that every day we kept the baby in was a huge achievement for which we were thankful. Tommy stayed with me for an early dinner together and he left to go get some sleep. He made sure his phone was on loud just in case anything happened through the night and told me to just keep calling as he was terrified he would sleep through a phone call. We said goodnight and both went to bed early.

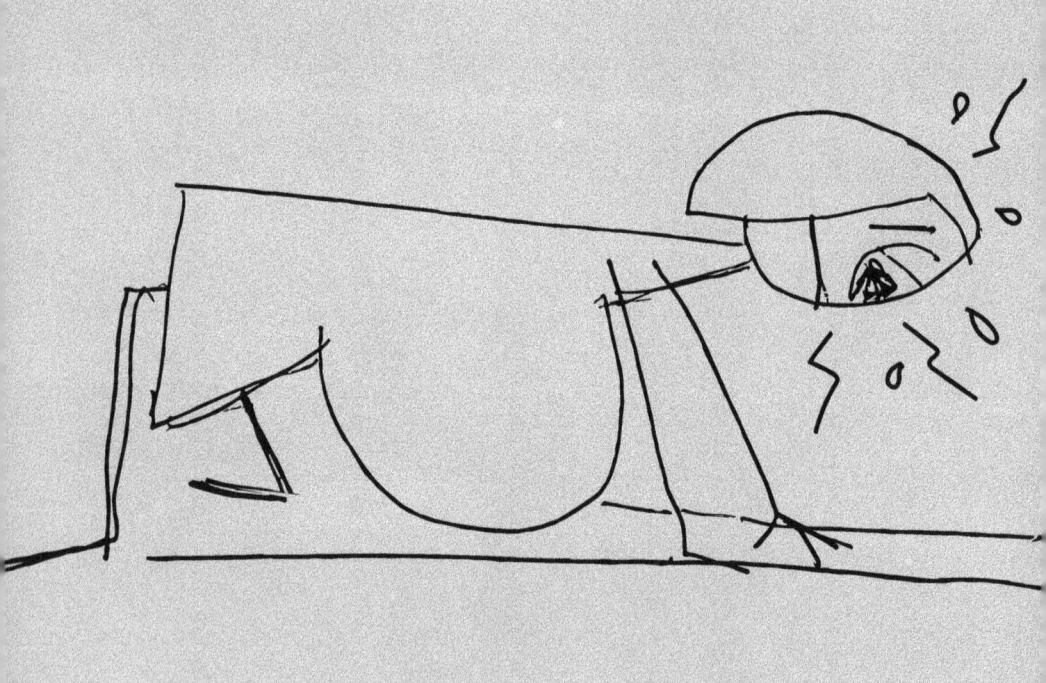

SOMEONE WAS WATCHING OVER US

THE FEMALE BODY is beyond incredible, and I am forever in awe of its power. I remember this moment so clearly. It was Friday 4th September, 2020. I woke up and looked at my watch – 1:17 am. I knew a midwife would be in soon to do OBS, so I tried to go back to sleep. Then I felt it. A huge gush of fluid. I sat up.

"No no no no no!" I yelled as I desperately and naively tried to regather the fluid and hold it all in. It was pointless. I sat there in a puddle of amniotic fluid which had saturated my pyjamas and the bed. I hit the buzzer for the midwife to come in and turned the light on.

In came a midwife and I said, "My waters have just broken everywhere.

She smiled and said, "That's okay, love. Let me get the bed cleaned up for you. You're about 34/35 weeks, aren't you?"

I looked at her and said, "Uhh no, I'm 24 + 3 today."

Her demeanour changed slightly, and she said she would get the registrar right away.

"I'm just going to go to the bathroom and clean myself up," I said.

She nodded as she contacted the registrar. After giving myself a bit of a wipe in the bathroom and getting changed, I came back out while the bed was still being made and sat on the chair off to the side.

The registrar was ready but needed me on the bed to have a look at my cervix. I lay back down on the bed as the young man bent down to put the speculum in. My waters were still gushing so he kindly said to me, "I can't see anything with your waters still coming out, so I'm going to have to do an internal. Is that okay?" I nodded and looked up at the ceiling. He gently put his fingers into my vagina. What he said next was never something that had even entered my mind.

"I've got a foot – get on your hands and knees!"

He pulled his hand out with urgency and I quickly flipped myself over onto my hands and knees with my head down and my backside high in the air. Yep, I had a foot hanging out of my cervix. My baby had busted my waters by shoving his foot through my cervix. COOL! I can't remember exactly what was said to me at this point, but I was rushed off to the birth suite with my ass in the air fully exposed, and I was madly trying to call Tommy to let him know I was being taken to theatre. There was no option for natural delivery – baby was footling breech, and given the size of him, if I didn't dilate quickly enough there was the possibility that his skull would be crushed on the way out, which would obviously result in death. Yeah, not an option.

Tommy answered on the second ring, and I calmly said, "My

waters broke and I'm waiting to be taken into theatre. You need to get over here quick."

I was kept in the birth suite for a very short amount of time and willed myself to remain calm. All of my calm birthing techniques came flooding back and big deep breaths kept me from completely losing my shit. Keep in mind, all the while my bare backside is still on show. I remember thinking how ironic it was that I was stuck in this position. For any birthing woman, your dignity goes completely out the window, and you couldn't care less what is on show. At the time, I didn't even notice that my backside was exposed as I was too busy concentrating on my breathing. I do recall a midwife saying, "Do we think we could get a sheet for this woman to cover her up a little bit?" A sheet was then draped over me.

Within what felt like seconds after I hung up the phone with Tommy, he appeared in the birth suite huffing and puffing.

Now, a little side story. On his road trip to this hospital, Tommy had stopped at a service station and purchased himself a pair of cheap thongs as he had forgotten to pack any. The previous day, he had shown me how many blisters they had given him and when I suggested he get some band aids he said to me, "Nah, I'm just going to man up and deal with them. They'll be right!" As I was currently on all fours, I was pretty much staring at his feet. After sprinting over to the hospital in these shitty thongs, he arrived all busted and bleeding from every single blister and his feet looked a mess. He was smart enough to read the room and realise it was not the time to be complaining about busted blisters!

As I have mentioned before, I have a lot of anxiety letting any old doctor operate on me. I can't recall the circumstances at this point, but Tommy and I were separated here, and I had thought he wasn't allowed in the room for the birth due to Covid restrictions. I stayed on all fours and continued my deep breathing as I was wheeled into theatre, praying that this young doctor who had examined me earlier would do a good job and wouldn't let me or the baby die. I was told I could lie on my back while the anaesthetist inserted the cannula into my hand, and out of nowhere up popped Dr F (the MFM).

A wave of relief flooded over me, and I knew we would be okay. He explained to me that due to the size of my uterus at such an early gestation, he would be performing a classical caesarean section, which meant that on the outside I would be cut horizontally, but on the inside, I would be cut vertically. This also meant that should we not require a hysterectomy and I was able to keep my uterus, I would never be able to deliver vaginally again. Quite frankly, I didn't care at this point.

I was sat up in theatre so that the anaesthetist could insert the blocker into my spine, and as I looked around the room I saw people everywhere. My legs began to tremble with anxiety as I tried my best to hold still. One of the theatre nurses clearly noticed and he came up beside me, put his arm around me and gently reassured me that everything would be okay; he said that I was in great hands and I was doing a great job. He was a big burly man with tattoos on his arms and a beard under his mask. It's people like this that you need in theatre rooms. I will never forget him. As my legs continued to shake, he put his hand on my knee to hold it still and gently reminded me to hold as still as possible for the needle to go into my spine. I was so thankful he was there. Theatre rooms can make you feel invisible, as if you are just another procedure, not a person; and this man made me feel safe without even trying. That is exactly what an incredible nurse does.

The needle was in, and I was laid down flat as the big blue screen was placed between my head and the rest of my body. This all happened quickly. At 2:15am, Tommy suddenly appeared beside me in theatre and was happy to see me so calm. I could hear one of the nurses say to him, "She is amazing. We can't believe how calm she has been." On the inside I was terrified, and I think this was about the time when I left my body and hit autopilot. It was as if I floated up above the room and was watching everything from above.

Having a C-section is a bizarre feeling. I could feel what I could only explain as "rummaging" around. At 2.22am I heard Dr F state time of birth and we heard the tiniest little squeak from our baby. Dr F quickly said, "Look, look!" He showed us the tiniest baby we had ever seen and handed him off to the NICU staff to intubate him. I stayed calm. I just felt this odd sense of "everything will be okay – we are both going to be okay". While Dr F continued to work on me and my placenta, Tommy was allowed to cut the cord. Our baby boy was born a tiny 700g (just under 1lb 9oz) and 32.5 cm long.

I lay there patiently waiting to get a glimpse of our baby and honestly, I can't really remember it. I have seen photos and watch videos of that moment when the wonderful NICU nurses presented our baby boy to us and explained what they were going to do and where they were taking him, but I can't physically remember it. As I said, I had left my body by this point. In the video from this moment, I am tearily saying thank you to the NICU nurse holding our baby close enough for me to kiss his head. With that, he was whisked away to be cared for and Tommy went with him.

Dr F popped up beside me and explained that my placenta had come away very easily, and he was able to clean out my uterus while he was there. He was hopeful that this meant the scarring would not return and that I would soon be transferred into recovery. While I was stitched back up, I remember trying to picture our baby's face. When we found out he was a boy, we had two names picked out ready to go, both of which did not suit him whatsoever once I saw him. For some reason, the name "Harry" immediately had popped into my head when I looked at him. He just looked like a Harry. This was not a name Tommy and I had discussed with any of our pregnancies.

I waited in recovery and at this point, still couldn't feel the pain from the surgery. The lovely nurse explained to me that she would give me some Endone and once I was able to have something to eat and drink, I could go back to the ward. Tommy appeared and told me our little boy was all settled in, and they would be able to wheel me past his room quickly before I could have a rest.

"What do you think for a name?" Tommy asked me.

"The two we have don't suit him at all, I don't think," I said to Tommy.

"What do you think of the name Harry?" he asked.

I stared at him dumbfounded. "You know, when that nurse held him by me to kiss his head, I instantly thought he looked like a Harry. How the hell have we both thought of that name without even talking about it?"

We didn't settle on Harry right away – I wanted to look at him again before we decided to name him. But I think we both knew that was already his name.

It was the early hours of the morning and my mother and father were on the road, bringing Addie to visit us. Tearful messages were exchanged between Mum and me when I told her I'd had the baby. Tommy had messaged her earlier letting her know I was being taken to theatre, but she hadn't realised I had already had him. I was excited to see Addie later that afternoon, not realising how much pain I would be in.

The Endone suddenly kicked in and quite frankly, I felt like a bag of dicks. I started sweating profusely, trying not to vomit, and my whole world was fuzzy. I felt so completely out of it that I don't even remember seeing Harry on my way back to the ward. I vaguely recall Dr F coming in to see me, seeing how sweaty I was and ordering immediate antibiotics, as he was concerned I had developed an infection. I begged the midwife to not give me any more Endone as I felt so sick and knew I just needed to sleep it off a bit. The anaesthetic had completely worn off by this point and I was in a lot of pain.

Tommy decided to go back and get some sleep as well and came in to hug me, forgetting that I had just been completely sliced open, and he leant right on my belly. I nearly spewed. Finally, I was left alone to concentrate on not dying from the effect Endone had on me, and try to sleep it off.

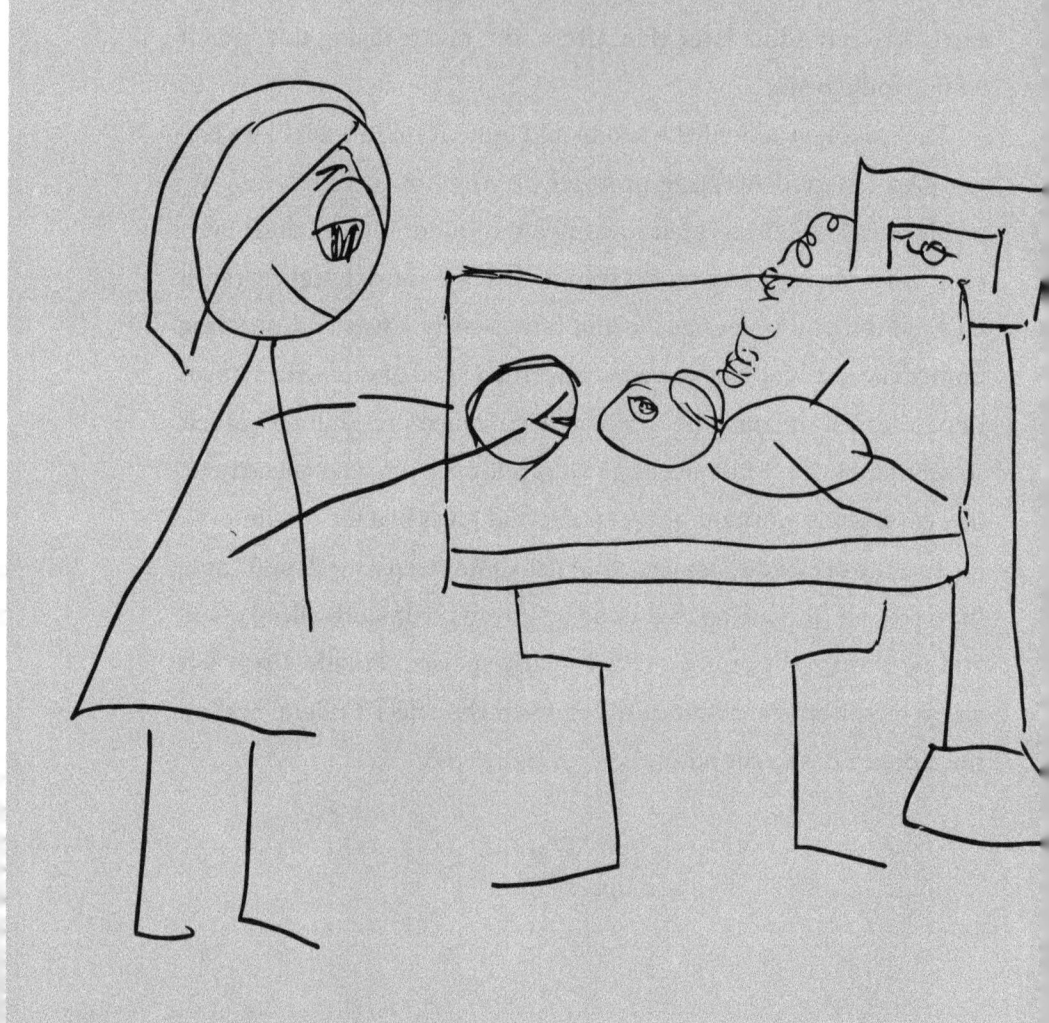

ADJUSTING TO OUR NEW NORMAL

I WAS WOKEN by a midwife a few hours later, who told me it was time to get up and get moving. She was going to help me shower. I had a drain poking out of my pubic area, which had a bag attached to it for excess blood. I was in a lot of pain trying to move but I willed myself to get to the shower, as I could smell my dried sweat from my earlier Endone episode. I stank!

We managed to get me into the shower, and thank God there was a chair in there because the young midwife kindly said, "Okay, I'm just going to sit you down for a minute and get you a sick bag; you're a lovely shade of green." I could feel it too. I felt as if I'd been on a spinning ride for far too long and the whole world was still going around way too fast for me. I gripped onto the chair as hard as I could and closed my eyes. The warm water on my back felt amazing. Thankfully, I didn't end up needing to vomit, my colour came back, and my world stopped spinning. I was able to wash myself and feel half human again before being helped back into a standing position, dried, clothed, and escorted back to my bed. After my awful reaction to Endone, I would only accept Nurofen and Panadol as pain relief. I'm pretty sure they did nothing, but it was worth a try.

I have never been an advocate for birthing any other way other than what is right for you, your body, your baby and your situation. Since I have now had both a vaginal and a C-section birth, I can honestly say that I would rather birth vaginally every single morning just to kickstart my day, over ever having a damn C-section. C-section mothers are warriors. I was still in pain at 11 weeks post-partum, and to this day I have serious sensitivity on my scar. One thing I had not prepared myself for were the afterbirth pains. They were no joke! I swear, after having full-blown contractions you hardly even notice the afterbirth pains. After my C-section, the afterbirth pains were so full on that at one point I was seriously considering asking if I could hang off the gas for a few hours.

Tommy returned in the afternoon, after we'd both had a bit more sleep, and the staff organised a wheelchair for me to go and visit our baby boy. At this point I had never felt so heavily reliant on Tommy; he had to physically help me out of bed and into a wheelchair, then grab my super fashionable blood bag and hook it onto the wheelchair. Real cute. The way to keep the mystery alive in a marriage! I was in so much pain that even going over tiny bumps in the wheelchair nearly made me spew.

Tommy and I had decided that we would name our little boy after spending a little more time with him. I was wheeled into NICU, down a corridor and into a little room where our baby lay in an incubator with wires and leads everywhere, and machines beeping noisily. To say it was surreal is an understatement. I don't remember much from this visit; I was able to take one photo of him before I started to feel extremely hot and dizzy. A NICU ward is generally quite warm and given that I was still feeling pretty sick from the Endone, I started to feel really faint. I told Tommy I needed to go back to bed, so he quickly took me back to the maternity ward.

After some umming and ahhing, we settled on the name Harry. For some reason, every time we both looked at him, we just kept seeing him as a Harry. All the Harrys we had known were complete ratbags, and we both felt that ours would be no different. I was able to get a bit more of a sleep before our daughter was brought in to visit. I was so happy to see and hold her, and she was really gentle with me. We were lucky that she understood that Mummy had "owies" and she had to be super careful and gentle. She looked at photos of her brother and somehow comprehended that we now had "baby Harry" in our lives, even though it would be an extremely long time before she would be able to meet him.

I don't intend on going into too much detail on our NICU journey with Harry. That would potentially be an entire book in itself. Tommy and I made the tough decision to send Addie back with my parents so she could continue going to daycare and have some sort of normalcy at least for the first few weeks, as we didn't know what was going to happen. I can remember telling Tommy that if Addie was with us and we got a call in the middle of the night from the hospital telling us that Harry wasn't going to make it, I didn't want to have to make the heartbreaking decision about who got to go and say goodbye to Harry while the other stayed with Addie. It just didn't bear thinking about. We knew that until Harry reached at least the 27/28-week mark, it was touch and go.

It was a heart-wrenching decision for us to make, and I remember the morning she left so clearly. I woke at about 2.30am, still in hospital and knowing my mother would be collecting a sleepy Addie from Tommy to get most of the drive out of the way while she slept, and I lay there and cried. Even as I write this, the pain of it is still so fresh in my memory that tears are forming in my eyes. Horrible. We are so lucky that we have such supportive family, who were able to do this for us; but it didn't make it any easier on our hearts.

Tommy came up early that morning to lie with me in hospital. We both felt broken. What was worse was that we didn't know how much longer we would have to live our life this way – so separated. Having a 24-weeker means you don't leave hospital quickly, and in some cases, some families don't get to leave with their baby at all. We had to take one step at a time and lean on each other as much as we could.

Day 3 post-partum, I was discharged from the ward and was able to stay with Tommy in Ronald McDonald House, across the road from the hospital. Thankfully a wheelchair was organised, as walking even 200 metres was still a huge effort for me. Tommy was so excited to have me out of hospital that he completely forgot how much pain I was in, and basically sent the wheelchair at high speed over the blistered pavement that you find either side of a pedestrian crossing. Once again, I nearly spewed from the pain. He apologised profusely and then said, "I'm sorry, I'm just so excited to have you back with me!"

For the next few weeks, I needed Tommy to help me shower and get dressed and undressed; he cooked for me and made sure I had plenty of good food for my milk supply and loads of water as well. He did all the washing, made sure I napped as often as I could, and ran my milk over to Harry multiple times a day. I was expressing every three hours morning and night, which was exhausting. My breastfeeding journey with Addie was awful, but I knew Harry needed my milk to help him survive.

Breastmilk works more as medicine rather than food for such small babies, and I was determined that he would only get my milk to help him. In saying that, I am not one of these lucky women who can just connect themselves to a pump and have milk flooding out. I had to sit and do one breast at a time and use compression for the entire pumping session, massaging the milk out of my boobs. Even doing this, I would get only small amounts; and I developed such severe RSI in my thumbs and wrists from so much massaging that I nearly couldn't use my hands without being in pain. On top of this, when I was discharged from the hospital, I was given needles that I had to inject into my legs, to administer blood thinners to avoid developing clots. The bruising on both of my legs looked awful.

I was running purely on autopilot; my alarm went off every three hours around the clock, and I connected myself up to my pump and started my process. I ate the food Tommy placed in front of me three or four times a day, and we went to the hospital twice a day to do Harry's "cares", which involved wiping his eyes and mouth, nappy change and reposition. In between all this I would try to nap, desperately trying to recover from my surgery.

When Harry was five days old, I was allowed to have him placed in my hands whilst still in the incubator as his bedding was changed beneath him. Once again, I look back at these photos and I vaguely remember it happening, but I don't have any feeling that goes with it. I had completely shut myself down. I can remember telling myself to talk to him: do all the right things, make sure you touch and sing and chat away to him. He knows your voice. But I feel that having my baby plucked out of me at such an early gestation meant I hadn't fully connected with him in utero, so I found connecting with him on the outside incredibly difficult. I knew what I had to do so that he felt that connection and love, but I didn't actually feel it myself. It sounds horrible to say but sadly for me, it was the truth.

Harry was doing incredibly well and had remained nice and stable since birth. The nurses explained to us that his sats (blood saturation) kept swinging a bit all over the place, which meant they had to keep adjusting his oxygen requirements, but aside from that he was doing great. So, on Day 6, I was allowed to experience my first skin on skin (kangaroo care) with him. I can remember being really excited to hold him. It all happened in slow motion. He was lifted out by the incredible nurses and gently positioned on my chest. My gown was then wrapped around his little body and heated towels were placed over him. Immediately, his little body relaxed, the machines stopped beeping and his sats levelled out perfectly. I can remember the nurses asking if I could stay there 24/7, because he was clearly much happier on me than he was in an incubator. I cried as I was having my first little cuddle with him. My body knew he was my baby and flooded with love for him. It was a very overwhelming experience. This baby that could fit in the palm of my hands, that should still be in my belly, that I had to ask permission to hold, was now on my chest. His eyes were still fused shut, but he could feel me, and he obviously knew he was safe.

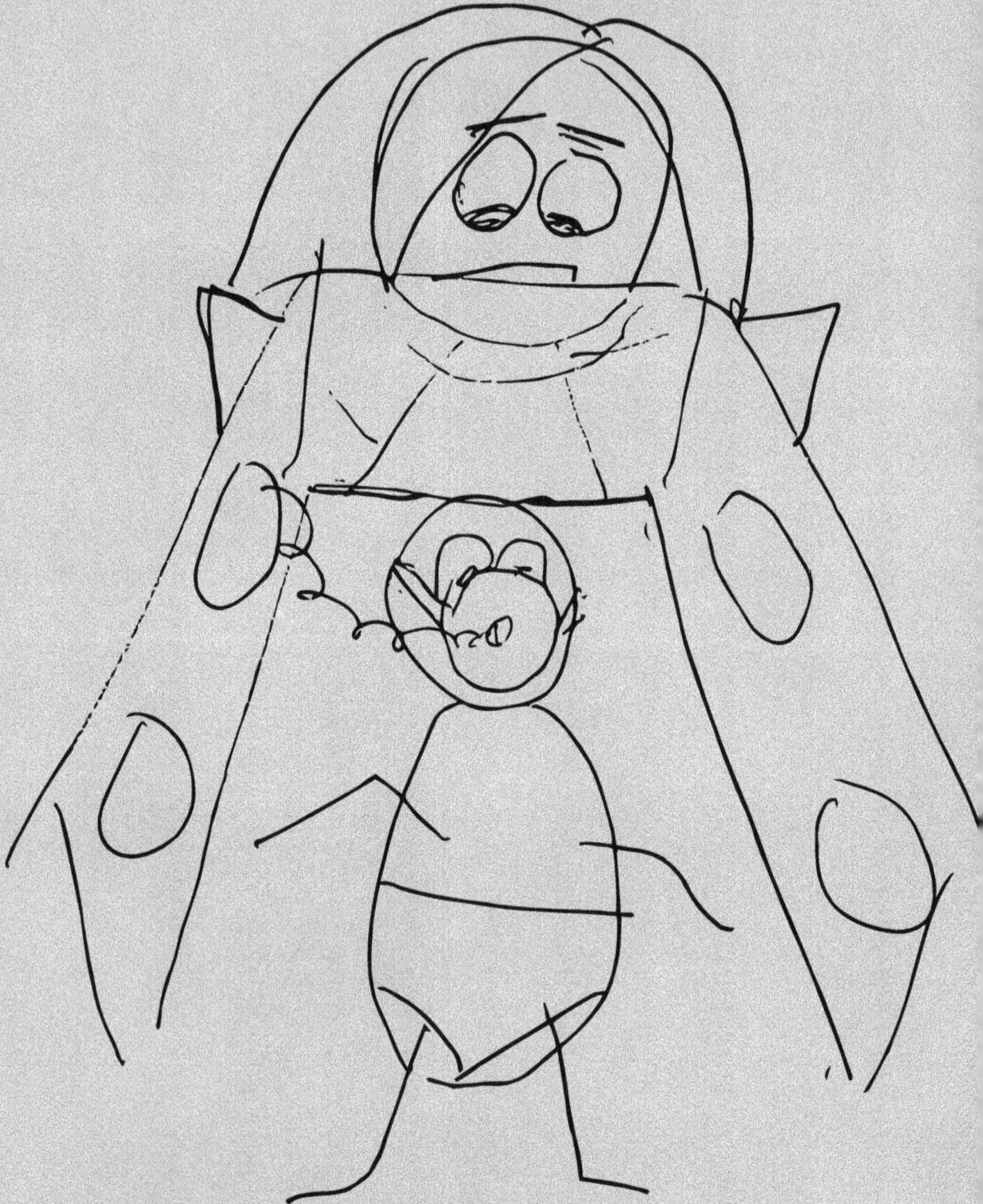

IT'S A JOURNEY

WE SPENT THE next thirteen weeks away from our home while our son remained in hospital. About two weeks after Harry was born, our families rallied together and all took turns in making sure someone was with us so that Addie could remain with us permanently in Ronald McDonald House. It meant we always had a third person available to care for her while we spent time at the hospital caring for Harry. Our days rolled into one as we got into a good routine keeping Addie busy and entertained for the morning. We would then visit Harry for his morning cares, come home for lunch, and Addie would have a sleep, then play time in the afternoon, before we went back up to Harry for his evening cares, then back home to put Addie to bed. It seemed as if we were there for a lifetime. Looking back on it now, that time was the easiest part of our journey. I would never wish it on anyone to have such an extremely premature baby; in saying that, being able to watch your baby grow, develop and fight to be alive was an absolute privilege.

Harry spent 93 days in this hospital. On 6th December 2020, Harry and I were transferred back to our home hospital via an RFDS flight. I remember that as the plane took off, my little baby and his oxygen tank beside me, the full magnitude of what we had achieved hit me all at once. I cried my eyes out watching the town where we had spent three months disappear below me. I had felt at home there; and the people around us, along with the friends we made, felt like home, a safe place. Outside the trauma of Harry being born so early, I also have many fond and happy family memories from this time. Given that I was so emotionally shut down, that is pretty much a miracle in itself.

The flight home was quite quick. We didn't land at the airport, but the aeroclub on the nearby tarmac. My father is a member of the aeroclub and often flies the light aircrafts for fun. As we pulled in, I could see him standing alone on the tarmac waiting. He is not really one for following rules, and I have no idea if he had been given permission to be there or not, but he knew the gate code to get onto the tarmac and he stood there waiting to see us briefly.

I should point out that I get quite motion sick – like, debilitatingly sick. I knew I had to keep it together to make sure Harry got settled into the Special Care Nursery in our home hospital, but by this point I didn't feel great.

My dad got a brief look at Harry and said, "Shit, he's little!" Thanks, Captain Obvious. He is actually huge now, but yeah, to anyone else he would look little.

There was a mix-up with the ambulance transfer so when one finally arrived, it was with two lovely young women who were from another town and had no idea what level to escort us to in the hospital. I willed myself to keep it together to direct both the flight nurse and the two ambulance officers with my precious cargo to the correct level. We finally made it into the special care nursery. I texted my dad to ask him drop me some Red Rooster and a bottle of Coke. I needed hot salty chips and Coke to settle my sickness.

I sat on a couch close to Harry and listened as the nurses did handover, providing whatever additional information I could. I thanked the RFDS flight nurse and the two ambulance officers for getting Harry here safely, and the special care nurses got Harry settled in. It was then that I completely fell apart. It was as if my body knew that Harry was here safely, and all the motion sickness that I had been trying to suppress hit me like a ton of bricks. I could feel how pale I was and was desperately trying to breathe through the feeling of wanting to spew.

"Are you okay?" one of the nurses asked me.

"I get really bad motion sickness. I'm fine. Just look after Harry and ignore me," I managed to get out. I can barely even speak when I'm that motion sick. I suddenly felt a cool face washer over my forehead, which was amazing.

I knew I needed to lie down in a dark room in peace. I desperately texted my family through half an open eye, asking for someone to come and pick me up because I was so sick I basically couldn't see. My oldest sister said she would be in the pick-up zone in five minutes, so I told the nurses I needed to leave and said I would return in the afternoon or early evening to sort Harry out; I knew he was safe now. With blurry eyes I stumbled out of maternity ward into an elevator and got to the pick-up zone as quickly as I could. Thankfully there was an empty chair, so I sat there slumped over with my face buried in my knees, waiting for my sister to arrive. She pulled up, and I dived in and just said, "Can't talk, I'm dying." She drove me around the corner to her house and let me die in her bed. I hadn't seen her for months so I'm well aware of how rude it was, but thankfully she understood and just sorted my life out around me.

I have no idea how long I slept, but she came into the room a while later and woke me up.

"Here are your boob tablets, and Mum said you have to express."

I wanted to tell her to fuck off. But feeling less than average, I sat myself up, took my Domperidone and connected myself to my pump. With the travel and craziness of the day, I hadn't expressed in almost eight hours, so my boobs were super full.

I finally recovered from my motion sickness and was able to get back up to the hospital with fresh milk and help to feed Harry. Tommy had spent the day on the road driving home with Addie, so I wanted to make sure I got home before they arrived. I bid Harry goodnight and made my way home. They made it home a short time after, and Addie was really excited to be back in her own bedroom with all her toys. It was amazing to be back in our home after a long three months.

※ ※ ※

We remained in our home hospital for two weeks and on the 15th December 2020, after 103 days in hospital, we were finally discharged with our baby boy. Harry was to remain on home oxygen 24 hours a day, until such time that he was able to pass an overnight respiratory assessment where he didn't desaturate. We had oxygen bottles installed in the house and were given a few travel tanks for when we had to leave the house. It was a strange feeling bringing Harry home. I had shut down so much of myself and completely detached from him, and I felt as if someone just handed me a baby and told me to love it. Obviously, in hindsight, my postnatal depression was there; and little did I know, it was only going to get worse. Much worse.

For many people, myself included, once a premature baby is home and out of hospital, it is assumed that everything is now okay. In our case, that was an absolute joke. Harry came with many challenges outside the oxygen requirement – challenges that took me to some dark places. I was adamant he had a tongue tie and reflux, and after a few weeks of trying to convince myself that wasn't the case, I got medication for his reflux and it definitely helped with the screaming. Harry was also a projectile vomiter. I'm talking exorcist-style vomiting where so much pressure built up behind it, he could shoot his vomit almost two metres across the room. For a tiny human, that is huge.

After being home with Harry for almost ten weeks and struggling to feed him with both breast and bottle, along with another four rounds of mastitis, I made the decision to get his tongue tie lasered. I needed improvement. I was doing daily physio with Harry; and I had seen speech therapists and dieticians who were stumped at the way I had to try and force-feed him. It was as if this baby had underdeveloped cheek muscles and physically couldn't suck. A baby that can't suck! WHAT? I would have to keep Harry moving whilst trying to feed him, to distract him from the fact that I was forcing a bottle into his mouth against his will. I then had to hold the bottle between my first finger and middle finger while simultaneously squeezing his cheeks together with my thumb and ring finger, and use my pinky finger to stimulate under his chin. This combination together meant he would feed, but it would take over an hour to get his feed in.

I also had to wake him through the night to try and get enough fluid into him. The dream feed is supposed to be the nicest one. Yeah. Not for Harry and me. I would fight him through the night because he didn't want it, but I knew he had to have it. Just keeping this baby hydrated was a battle that I fought every single day, and twelve-plus months on, I was still fighting daily with him for hydration.

It is so easy to look at someone and assume they are doing a wonderful job without actually taking into consideration the lengths to which they are going just to keep their child alive. We tried so many different things. I was told by different speech therapists that basically there was nothing else they could suggest, and I just had to keep battling away as I was and hope that once he was on solids, he would be more willing to take fluid and stop vomiting as severely. On top of the fighting to keep him hydrated, he would power spew multiple times a day. That was disheartening for me; we would have fought so hard to get a decent amount of fluid into him, only for him to spew it back up. I'm not sure people believed me when I described his spewing. One day, I was showing a speech therapist and dietician how I had to feed Harry, and I suddenly knew he was about to spew. I quickly shoved my chair out of the way and said, "Get back, it's coming!" Within seconds a pressure fountain of vomit came out of Harry's mouth and went right across the room. The two women sat there, eyes wide with shock and their jaws on the floor, and both just said, "Wow."

Let me be clear here. We tried everything. Every single thing that was suggested to me, I gave it a crack. I tried different teats for bottles, I tried having other people feed him, I tried cup feeding, syringe feeding; all the suggestions I was given, I tried. I just loved it when someone would say to me, "Just give him a sippy cup." It used to take all my strength not to come out with some smart-arse remark along the lines of "if it was that easy, fuckface, I would have done it by now"! I was angry. And I was getting angrier by the day.

I started to build up so much anger towards Harry for (1) taking me away from Addie, and (2) making it so hard just to keep him alive. Had I not been through enough? I mean, come on. He shoved his foot through my cervix at 24 weeks and he was still giving me a hard time. I know, I know; it wasn't his fault. But when you are in a hole as dark as I was in, all you see is the problem in front of you and what/who is causing it. It can start to get dangerous.

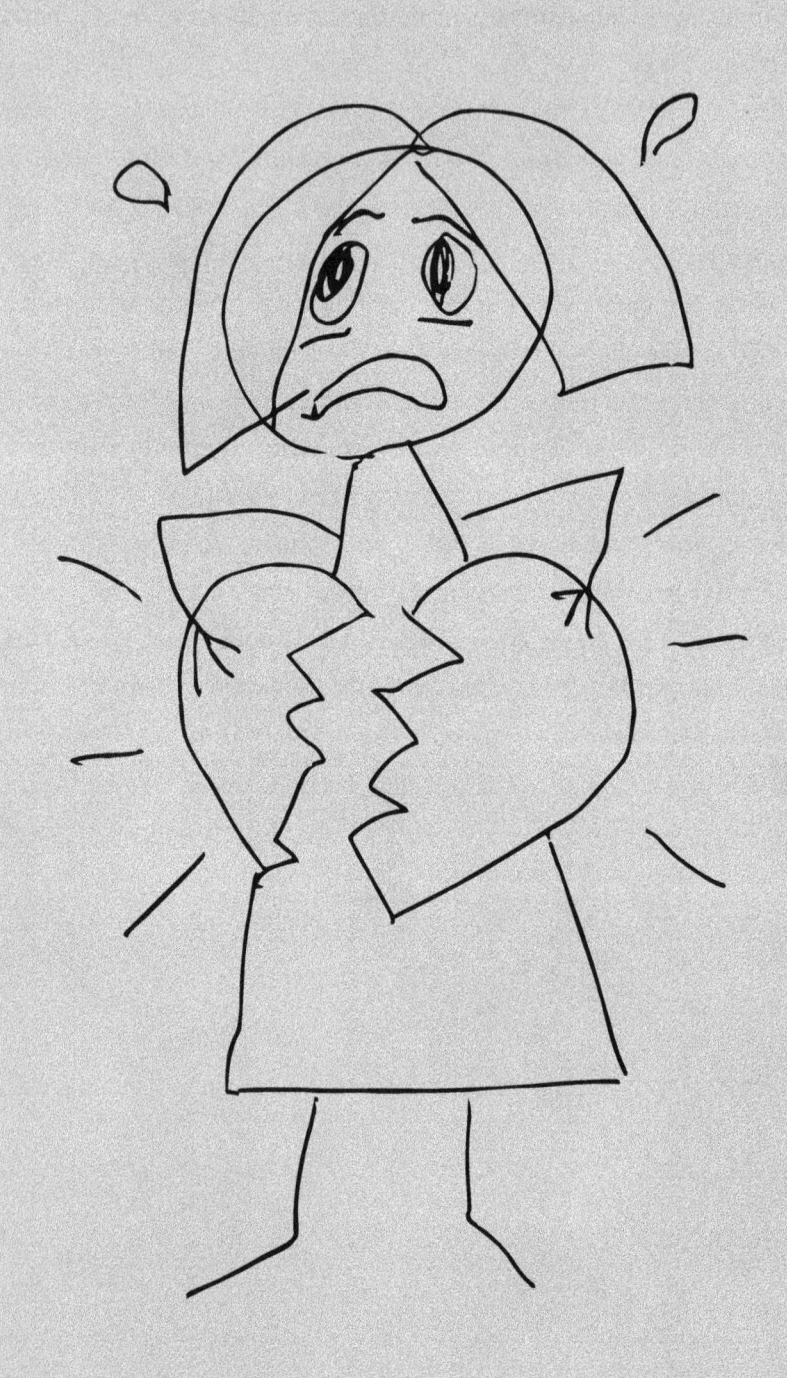

2021: THE WORST YEAR OF MY MENTAL HEALTH LIFE

I HAVE COME to realise that I have a way of presenting myself to the outside world, somehow playing down what is going on inside of me. It's something I am working on. 2021 was one of the darkest years I have ever endured. No one seemed to understand what I was dealing with, and every single person I talked to told me how amazing I was, that I'd been through so much, and I was so strong. Meanwhile, behind closed doors, I was wishing for some pretty horrendous things. I was also a very scary mother to both of my children; and quite frankly, I was scary to myself. I did not fit the "depressed" mould because I could still see and feel joy in my days. I still laughed, and I could still see the funny side of things. But there was something dark in me. Something that would explode over the silliest things. My mind would also tell me to do some truly awful things. I never did, and I am so very thankful that part of my logical brain was still able to operate. But damn, shit got scary sometimes.

I know there are people who have it worse than anything I have had to deal with. In no way am I trying to take away from what other people have been through. Trauma is trauma, and everyone deals with things completely differently. For me, this whole journey was extremely traumatic, and it made me angrier and more resentful as time went on. I can remember one time when I was sitting on the couch in my house after screaming at Addie for something. Harry was screaming, and there was still his fresh spew on the ground. I looked around at it all, looked at my kids and thought, "These kids would be better off without me." I started to think of ways I could make that a reality.

Other days, I just wanted to be by myself for a few months, so I started to think of ways that I could possibly get away with hurting Harry too, so that we would end up on separate wards in the hospital and I might get a decent break. I would fantasise about running the car into a tree when I had both kids in the car. I would look at power poles and think, *Now. Do it now.* It was usually while they were screaming in the back seat, and I just couldn't take any more.

I am being totally honest about these heinous intrusive thoughts I was experiencing, but I never acted on them, and I never hurt my children. There were absolutely times I came close, and I would recognise the danger and end up sending Harry to my mother for weeks at a time. I would get more sleep when I was not doing the night feeds, and it would be enough to top my bucket up with a tiny bit of patience and energy to try again. I busted my butt to build a connection with Harry; and I fully knew I was the problem, not him. Through all of this, I was somehow able to make people believe I wasn't nearly as bad as I truly was.

What concerns me the most, though, is how often a health professional will validate what you feel and tell you, "You've been through so much," but not actually hear what you are saying. I hate that statement "you've been through so much." It pisses me off. I know how much I've been through; I lived it! Three months after getting Harry home, I contacted my therapist and we discussed everything in depth. The problem here was, I can talk about my shit with anyone and everyone. If you want to hear about it, I will tell you every last little detail; I don't feel sad or overwhelmed or emotional when I talk about anything I have been through in my life. But it meant that talk therapy was basically a bit of a waste of time for me. I didn't realise it at the time, and I absolutely LOVE my therapist. However, I wasn't getting better – just, perhaps, getting better at hiding it or reassuring myself that "it was all in my head".

I took myself to my GP in April 2021 in the hopes of getting medication, because I was not improving. After telling me I had been through a lot (I damn well knew that), she booked blood tests for me, to make sure there wasn't any hormonal issue that we had missed. My bloods came back perfect and after my GP went through everything with me to tell me everything looked completely normal, my dumbfounded response was, "Great. So I'm just fucking crazy, then?"

She laughed and said, "Fiona, you *have* been through a lot. It is perfectly normal to feel like this. See how you go and if you still feel this way in a few months, then please come back and see me. Keep up with your therapist also."

I walked out feeling like an idiot and questioning everything I was feeling. This certainly didn't *feel* normal. I wasn't liking feeling like a psychopath or visualising killing myself and my children every time I got behind the wheel. It didn't feel normal to be screaming over insignificant things, or to have one slight inconvenience that completely ruined my day, and then be unable to shake off the cranky, angry feeling.

I want to be clear here. When I started this chapter, I mentioned that I have a way of presenting to the outside world a very different representation of what is going on inside. It was the fault of neither my therapist nor my GP, that they didn't pick up the severity of my postnatal depression. I was able to make them believe that yes, I was having a tough time and having some bad thoughts that I truly believed I would never act on, but we were all surviving. The truth is, we were surviving but I was having a hell of a tough time with it and couldn't understand why I felt so much rage pumping through my body.

Every day was hard. I struggled to get out of bed, but I did. I struggled to put a face on to the world when I had to show up to multiple appointments each week with Harry, but I did. I found it difficult to be happy for other people, show up at family events, or even give a shit about other people's lives. But I did it. Every single night, I would fall into bed at about 7.30pm in an absolutely exhausted state, only for my alarm to go off a few hours later so I could get up and force-feed Harry through the night, then start the same process all over again the next day.

I wasn't getting better. In fact, I was getting worse. I had finally come to a place where I was eating healthily, sleeping well, and exercising daily. I did this religiously for five weeks straight and yes, I felt really good about my body. My head, though – my head was going into a downward spiral. Suicidal thoughts became more frequent,

I was getting angrier with both kids, and I was pushing my body to new limits just trying to exercise the anger out of me. It was useless. There was one day when I had so much built-up anger, I went for a run and just kept running. I ended up running 12 kilometres. And while I felt a bit mellowed out by the time I got home, that all too familiar bubbling of anger would come flooding back to me and I would explode. When I finally broke down to Tommy and let him in on what I had been feeling, he moved mountains to get me to a doctor and support me in needing medication. Through no fault of his own, he'd had no idea it was as severe as it was.

Tommy is amazing at making me laugh when I don't want to. From the stories in this book, you can tell he is a beautiful man. I'll never forget his support during one of the darkest times in my life, and the look on his face when he realised how serious I was about wanting to leave this earth. I managed to get an urgent appointment with my GP, and I begged her for medication. She arranged for a script of Sertraline to be collected and Tommy was able to pick it up for me the following afternoon on his way home from work. I just wanted to feel happy. Logical me was able to look at my life and realise how lucky I was. I had a loving and caring husband, we had a great house, were financially stable, had two beautiful children who were both happy and healthy, and we had a fantastic support system around us and wonderful friends who continued to reach out all the time. So why wasn't I happy? It made no sense to me. I felt broken. Completely defeated by own mind.

It didn't take long for the medication to start working. I felt amazing! The moment I knew it was working was when I was trying to feed Harry some puree and Addie was playing beside me with a soft toy. I had asked her to stop flinging it around while I was feeding Harry, in case she accidentally knocked the food out of my hand. What do you think happened? As I directed a spoonful of sloppy puree towards Harry's mouth, Addie flung the toy and whacked the spoon out of my hand, and the puree landed with a splat across my forehead. She stopped, with a look of terror on her face, waiting for me to explode. Without even thinking about it I just started to piss myself laughing! She looked relieved and said, "Are you happy, Mummy?" I just pulled her in for a cuddle and asked her to help me clean up the mess on my face. It felt like I was back. This felt more like me. If this had happened the week before, I probably would have pegged the rest of the food and dragged Addie screaming to her bedroom and shut the door with a loud bang.

When Tommy came home that night, he said to me, "I feel as if we should have gotten you onto medication a long time ago. I honestly just thought this was what life was going to be like with two kids, and you'd just be a bit cranky for a few years. But I feel like I've got my mate back!" Without either of us realising it, he had been walking on eggshells, not knowing what would set me off on an angry rampage. To be fair, the fortnight before this I had abused him over corned beef. Corned beef! And he had just stood there staring at me and copped it on the chin. Yep. As I said, it was usually over very silly stuff.

The medication kicking in was a massive turning point for me. It was around this time, too, that I was able to think a bit more clearly about everything, and I felt patient enough to try more ways of feeding Harry. One of the dieticians had sent me a recipe for custard using Harry's formula. Tommy suggested that we make it quite thick, like his purees, and give him his milk feeds that way rather than fight him with a bottle. This turned out to be a game changer.

I don't intend to go too deeply into all of Harry's feeding issues, developmental delays, need for physio multiple times a day, etc. He was born at 24 weeks and for all intents and purposes, he is a happy healthy little boy. Just looking at him, you would never know the struggles that have gone on behind closed doors. Or the blood, sweat and tears it has taken to get this little boy to where he is today. I believe that if he wasn't born to such an intense mother, he would have ended up being tube or peg fed. There would have been nothing wrong with that; and there were days when I was desperate for that scenario to be our reality as it would have made feeding times a much more pleasant experience for both of us.

Once we moved to custard feeding and he wasn't exerting so much energy trying to fight me multiple times a day, his physical development progressed a lot more quickly. For quite some time, he was anywhere from 3-5 months behind his corrected age. That made it feel like we had a newborn for a long time; and unfortunately, I hate the newborn stage.

The day of Harry's first birthday arrived, and while I wasn't feeling particularly emotional in the lead-up to it, the morning of that day was a different story. Tommy and I got Addie out of bed, and we all went in to wake Harry and say happy birthday. I started crying as soon as we got into the room. Tears rolled down my face. This little boy had come so far in 12 months, and I was so damn proud of what we had achieved together; especially while I was battling such an overwhelming darkness.

I worked daily on developing my attachment and connection with Harry; and it fills my soul with happiness that he lights up so much whenever I enter the room. This little boy knows he is loved. So, for me, I've obviously done something right.

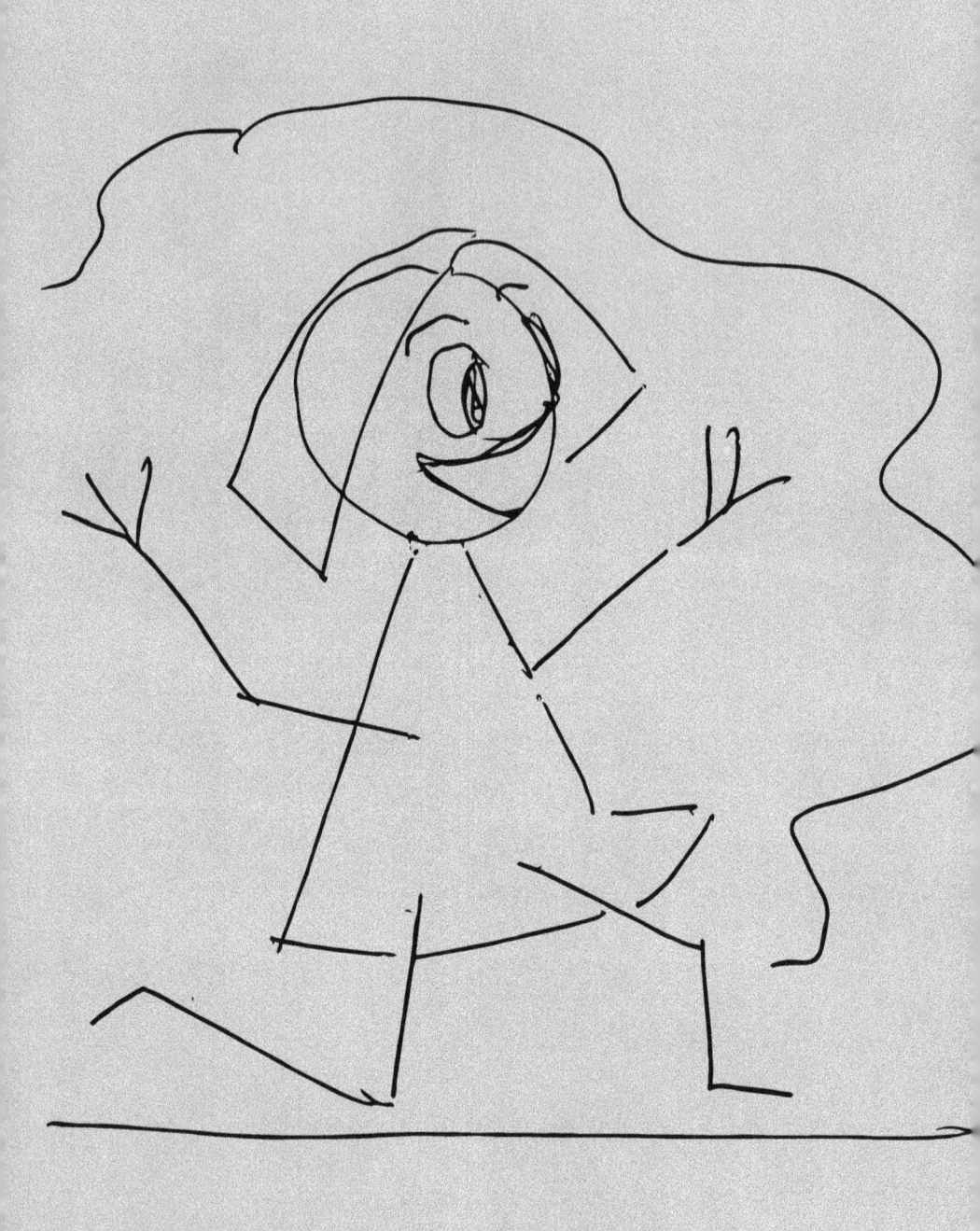

WHERE DOES THE STORY END?

BY THIS POINT, it was January 2022. The last few months of 2021 had been tough. My medication kept wearing off, so I would revert to feeling like a psycho and again have so much anger towards my life. I was referred to a psychiatrist and was put on the highest possible dose of Sertraline. I ended up seeking alternative therapies, as I firmly believe that for me, medication is a band aid, and I have some deep-rooted issues I needed to work through in order to get back to being me.

Medication certainly helped me realise that I didn't have to feel so awful all the time, and it opened my eyes to how it felt to be happy with your life and not permanently clouded by unnecessary and unwarranted anger. But unfortunately, with it continuing to wear off, the lack of consistency was extremely frustrating for both myself and my children. They didn't understand why Mum was happy, patient and loving one week, then a screaming banshee who didn't even want them around her the next. The important thing is, I don't want to be the latter, and I refuse to let this go on for the rest of our lives. It is no way for my children to live, and it's no way for me to live either.

People have asked me if I would have another baby. The young, broken mother in me who has lost so many babies would absolutely have more children. I would have ten more if I could. The realist in me, who has every teeny tiny trauma from the last six years physically engrained into my entire body, along with the woman who knows pregnancy after loss is terrifying let alone after what I've now dealt with, would not have any more children. I also never want to experience the post-partum hormonal dump and mental imbalance again. But it is a hard question to answer. I don't know what a future successful/viable pregnancy for me would even look like. I will never say never; however, our happy little family of four deserves all my love and attention for now.

Part of me longs for a stress-free pregnancy, a controlled birth, an easier newborn stage, and a baby that doesn't need so much of me. By that, I mean one that fits into the chaos without creating a whole new element of its own. Wishful thinking, I know. The first six months of both of my kids' lives were really tough on me. Whilst I felt so sad for how they must have been feeling through it all too, they won't remember it. I, however, will. I look back at photos of myself through those times and it breaks my heart to see how broken I look. My eyes always give me away. I can be smiling and look completely happy to everyone else, but I see the pain and anger. So much anger over having to constantly claw my way through really hard periods on every single level – physically, emotionally and mentally.

I am beyond fortunate that I have the family I have. We are all fairly dysfunctional in our own ways, but when it counts, we band together and help pick up the pieces of each other's problems. My own mother has created such a strong foundation of selflessness in myself and my two sisters, that when people show up in our own lives who need our support, we are there wholeheartedly. And for each other, even more so. I can't go on without highlighting how truly blessed I am for having the husband that I have. No relationship is perfect, and ours certainly has many cracks that we have both worked hard to repair. He is truly my best friend and biggest support system; he is more than willing to get amongst some of the weird and wonderful ways I have tried to heal myself, just so that I feel supported. Obviously, he likes to throw some friendly banter in there to stir me up, but it makes me very happy that he cares so much for my well-being.

There are many women across the country and around the world who have a similar story to mine, or one day will go through similar things. I hope this book gives an idea of what goes on behind closed doors, and what is beneath that happy smile and outgoing personality. Having a family is not easy, and when it is something you badly want, each let-down becomes more harrowing than the last. For me, the pain of loss grew into so much resentment and anger that when I finally did have successful pregnancies, I wasn't able to see how lucky I was. All I could see and feel was the anger that I was dealt such a tough hand. When you are in the throes of hardship, it's easy to get stuck there and feel as if there is no light at the end of the tunnel. That was me; I got stuck there. My brain has this awful way of only focusing on the negatives, regardless of how many positives there are in the scenario. It's something I'm working on.

As I mentioned earlier, I have started some alternative therapies to help me deal with my mental health. I started hypnosis therapy recently, and the first two sessions were focused on anger. The second session was incredible. It was like watching a movie of my memories on a big screen. First, we focused on all the memories where I had experienced the emotion of anger. Things popped up on this screen that I hadn't thought about in years; things I thought I had dealt with, but clearly, my subconscious hadn't let go. After going through all the memories where I had experienced anger, it was time to go back to the start and go through all the memories where I had experienced happiness. This, by far, was my favourite part. So many wonderful memories from my childhood through to now flashed across the screen; and all I could focus on was my big, happy smile. I can remember sitting there feeling as if I was going to cry. It was beautiful to be reminded of all of these happy moments that had somehow been suppressed under all of my negativity towards my life. Whenever I get low, or have a bad day, I picture this session and remind myself that yes, I have had a truly wonderful life, despite the few hiccups along the way.

A friend asked me recently, "So where does the story end?" I can't answer that. Maybe it never ends? My goal is to focus on bettering my mental health so that I can be a great and happy mother to my beautiful children who made it earthside. They were sent to me for a reason, and I intend to give them the best version of me moving forward. If I could change one thing about the last six years and everything I have been through, it would be the impact it has had on my mental health. Obviously, I would love to have had a simpler journey to parenthood, but I have been one of the lucky ones to be blessed with two children. Sometimes, you just have to be okay with how your story turned out, roadblocks and all. And I definitely am.

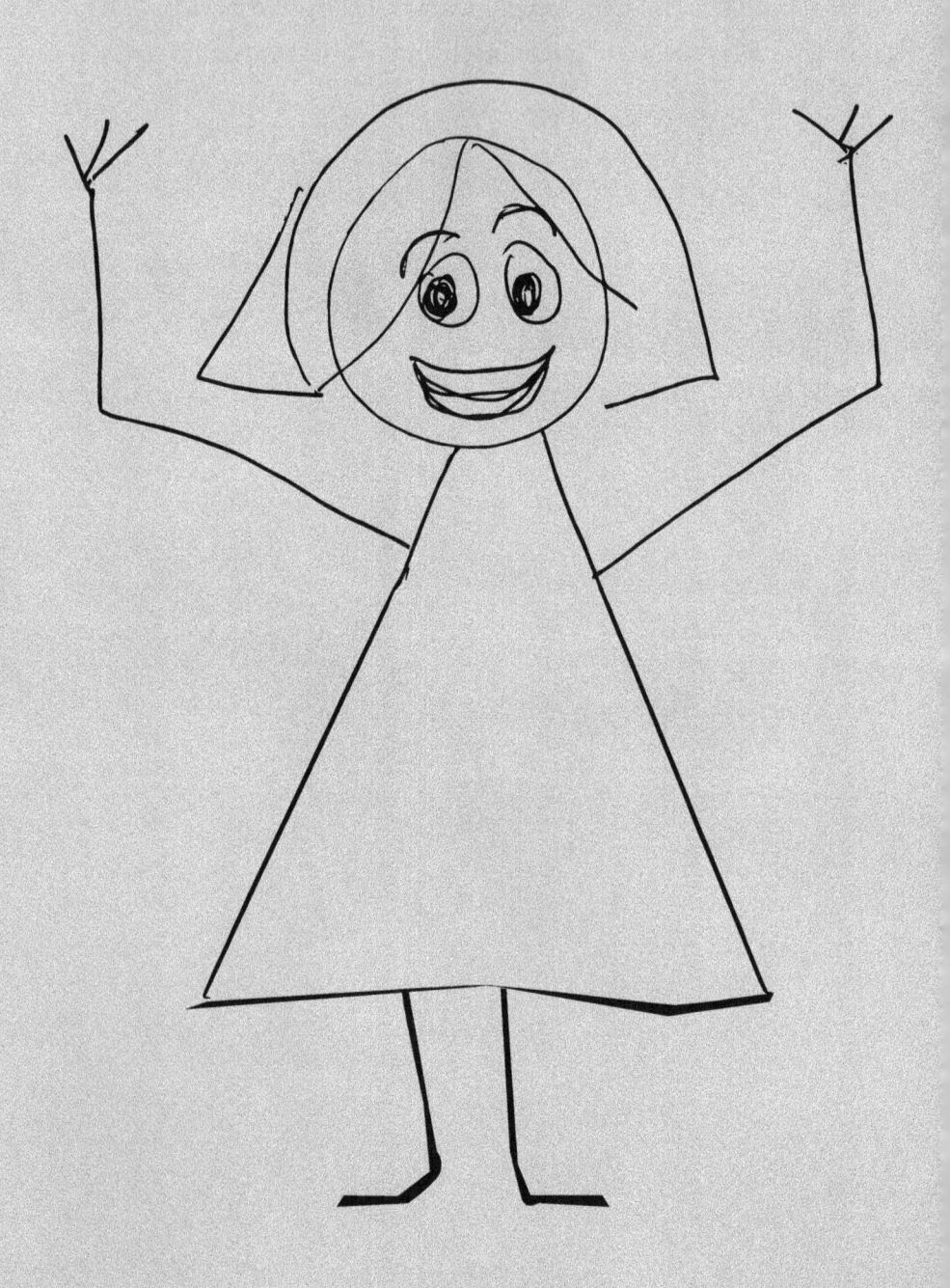

EPILOGUE

THE PREVIOUS CHAPTERS were completed in early 2022, and on the 6th of September that year, I got one hell of a positive pregnancy test. To say it was a shock is an understatement. When I found out, Tommy and I refused to speak to each other for approximately four hours. We both needed time to process what was happening. Tommy was the first to crack.

"It's going to be okay. We're going to have a third baby. I think I'm okay with it."

I could have strangled him. I was terrified.

We made it to 31 weeks with our second little man. Due to an additional complication with this pregnancy, my waters broke bang on 31 weeks + 1 day. Of course, it was pure chaos. My waters broke at approximately 10 pm. Similarly to what happened in both previous pregnancies, I woke out of sleep a few seconds before it happened and instantly knew. I flew out of bed saying out loud, "Okay, okay, okay!" as if trying to tell my waters not to make a mess on the carpet so I could reach the toilet. I was home alone with two sleeping children; Tommy was in Brisbane for work and my mother was in Byron Bay… greaaaaaaat.

I rang my middle sister and casually said, "So my waters have broken. I'm all good. I'm not contracting but obviously need to get to the hospital. Can you come over here and get the kids to daycare tomorrow so I can get to the hospital ASAP?" She graciously agreed and ended up bringing her husband with her so that he could drop me to the hospital on his way home. I rang Tommy, who was on a night out with his work friends, and when he saw my name show up on his phone so late at night he knew something was wrong.

"Hello?" he answered sternly.

Once again, me trying to be breezy. "Heyyyyy, babe, how's your night?" You know, small talk is key in moments like this.

"Yeah, good till you rang me. What's going on?" You could hear him sober up almost instantly.

"My waters have broken so I'm heading up to the hospital. Here we goooooo again!"

He did not share my sarcastic enthusiasm.

As I have said many, many times, pregnancy is a nasty business. I had been diagnosed with polyhydramnios, which basically meant I had a significant volume of amniotic fluid (more than is considered normal), so when I say I was gushing fluid, holy moley, was it coming out of me! I answered the door when my sister and her husband arrived with nothing but a towel between my legs because nothing else was soaking up the amount of fluid coming out of me. What a sight for my brother-in-law! Having had relatively stress-free pregnancies themselves, this was a whole new situation for them. I gave

EPILOGUE

my sister a brief rundown of what the kids would need the following morning, optimistically hoping that labour would be stopped and I could stay in hospital. I grabbed a few extra towels and a nightgown to give myself a tiny bit of dignity, and jumped in the car with my brother-in-law.

The poor bastard, seriously. "What's going on, Fi? Like, are you gonna have this baby in the car or what?" he asked nervously as I sat on two towels just casually leaking fluid.

I laughed at him. "No, I'm definitely not. I have a stitch in my cervix to keep it closed and I'm not in any pain, so I'm clearly not dilating. My waters just couldn't take the pressure of all the excess fluid. So you won't be delivering a baby in the car, dude."

You could see the relief in his eyes. We arrived at the hospital and he kindly walked me to the maternity ward. The 15-minute drive had meant I'd leaked through two towels and my nightgown, and I walked into the hospital with amniotic fluid running down my legs, leaving a trail behind me. Dignity? What dignity? That was long gone. Once I was put in a birth suite, the midwife didn't even need to check a pad, she could see it was amniotic fluid. I was put on a bed with CTG machines to check on bub, and administered Nifedipine to try and slow labour, as by this point I was getting tightenings that were taking by breath away.

Because I was 31 weeks, it meant I was unable to deliver in our home hospital and would need to be transferred. As with the situation with Harry, the major hospital that we were in the catchment for didn't have enough room, so was unable to accept my admission. Knowing that the hospital where I had Harry was unable to say no, I gently asked them to contact the NICU we had previously been to and to see if an RFDS flight was available for transfer there. While all of this was happening, my waters continued to gush out and at one point, a nurse had to come in and mop the floor beneath me. I had soaked through all the pads on the bed and was basically lying in a puddle that had started to overflow and spill onto the floor. I think I lost about four litres of fluid between my waters breaking and delivery. I was thrilled to find out the alternative tertiary hospital had accepted me, and that I would be sent on an RFDS flight by about 8am the following morning. I messaged Tommy and made sure he got a flight to meet me there, as it seemed that we would be delivering soon after arrival. I was so thankful, as it meant I would be with the same doctor who delivered Harry. Ahhhhhh, safety.

Right before I was transferred to the airport, the head of the Special Care Nursery came to see me. She happens to be a close friend of my mother, and she also helped me greatly through my journey with Harry. By this point, I hadn't even told Mum what was happening as I knew she was on the road driving and I didn't want to stress her out. So as soon as this woman walked through the door and gave me a big cuddle, I burst into tears. I had been fine up until this point. It suddenly felt as if, for a moment, someone else was able to be brave for me while I reset my nervous system and let it all out.

We made it onto the tarmac. Keep in mind I was STILL leaking by this point, and it was almost 12 hours since my waters had broken. The lovely flight nurse and doctor were desperately trying to keep my gown covering me while I was holding a towel between my legs and navigating all the cords that were attached to me, as well as the cannula in my hand.

EPILOGUE

"Don't even worry about it, ladies, just let go," I said. My care factor was well below zero and I didn't care who saw my bare backside as a gust of wind conveniently flew up under my gown. I just wanted to be able to get myself in the plane without the rank sensation of fluid uncontrollably coming out of me. They apologised profusely because there was a male pilot. To be honest, I felt sorrier for him then me.

The flight went smoothly and I was transferred via ambulance to the same hospital where we had spent three months with Harry. For most, this probably would have been a very scary and triggering moment. For me, I felt instant calm wash over me. We were in the right place and everything was going to be okay. Tommy met me at the door and we were sent into the birth suite to be monitored and for the doctors to make a decision on what to do. Tommy hadn't slept a wink and was still drunk from the night before, desperately trying to appear sober; ahhhh, it's an adventure.

By this point it was about 11am. I was exhausted as I'd been awake all night with all the monitoring and the disgusting gushing that meant I couldn't doze off. After a quick assessment, it was decided that they would schedule me in for surgery that afternoon at around 2.30pm, as they didn't want to risk my cervix dilating around the stitch I'd had put in place at 14 weeks in an effort to keep it closed. Knowing we had some time, Tommy and I both tried to get some sleep.

At about 12:30, a team of people burst into the room and said, "Sorry! We got the time wrong. It is actually 12.30 pm that you're scheduled, so we're off to theatre!"

I felt my entire body clench with fear. This was the part I was dreading. I knew the baby would be okay, but I had this underlying feeling that something would go wrong with me, and I was terrified.

I managed to keep it together as we were transferred down to theatre. As we were waiting for me to be put into a separate room to talk with the anaesthetist, my body started to shake. I started crying. The tears were rolling down my face. I didn't want to do this. Memories of the physical pain from Harry's birth started flooding back to me and I did not want to go through that again. What if I never came back out of this theatre? What if I never saw Addie and Harry again? What if Tommy had to watch his wife die? This was fucked. So many intrusive thoughts started to overwhelm me. Tommy quietly held me and kept telling me it was okay; we'd all be okay. I took some deep breaths and pulled myself together.

The anaesthetist was a lovely young guy who told me what he was going to give me. They had planned for a lower segment C-section which, given the size of the baby and my gestation, should be fine. I was thrilled that it would just be the bottom half of me being cut this time. I was wheeled into theatre and did my very best not to dissociate, and to take it all in. This was our last baby. I wanted to be present no matter what. Knowing I would have to have a C-section, I wanted to see the baby being lifted out of me. But because it was so early at 31 weeks, this was not an option. Thankfully, I realised part of the way into the procedure that I could see what was happening via the reflection of the stainless steel that was above me. I didn't see them cut me open as I was busy concentrating on not dying; whatever the anaesthetist had given me had started to make me boil and I was begging for cold towels over my face and neck. Once I had cooled down, I was able to intently watch the ceiling and wait for our baby to come out. We knew we were having another boy and I was excited to see him.

EPILOGUE

As if in slow motion, I watched the face of our little man come out of my belly in the reflection, and it was beautiful! I can't even put into words what a precious moment it was for me to see this. The doctor held our baby boy up and I grabbed the blue blanket they had blocking my belly and yanked it down so I could see him. He looked so big. Keep in mind the last baby that was pulled out of me was Harry, who was so very tiny. I looked at this little boy and thought, *You know, he looks ready to come home now.*

Charlie Thomas McBryde was born at 31 weeks + 2 days on 15/03/2023, at 1:56 pm, weighing in at 1.920kg. He was taken off to the Special Care Nursery as he seemed to be breathing okay, and Tommy went with him.

I felt relieved. I looked back up at the reflection of my stomach in the stainless steel and remember thinking that it looked like an absolute mess. I had a feeling things hadn't gone quite to plan. The doctor popped her head up beside me and explained that they had started with a lower segment C-section but every time they had tried to grab Charlie, he kept escaping. All that fluid he had to swim around in! They ended up having to do a repeat classical C-section – a horizontal incision on the outside and vertical incision on the inside.

"Okay," was all I managed to get out. I was devastated. I knew agony and a very long recovery was coming my way. To make matters worse, because it had only been planned for a lower segment to be completed and the procedure ended up taking much longer, the spinal block had started wearing off while they were still trying to sew me up. They were injecting local anaesthetic into my stomach while trying to stitch me up, but the internal pain I was starting to feel was becoming unbearable.

I have a pretty high tolerance for pain, as I've mentioned previously. But this pain was something else. As they were wiping my belly down after finishing up, it felt like they were whacking me with a baseball bat. It was excruciating. As they rolled me onto my side so they could lift me off the theatre table and onto a bed, I had tears rolling down my cheeks and I could hardly breathe through this pain. I was begging for pain relief. When I was sent into recovery, I was given Endone and it didn't even take the edge off. More and more Endone was given to me and I could feel it working in terms of me being bombed off my face, but the pain was not subsiding. Finally, I was taken back to the maternity ward and asked on a scale of 1-10 what my pain level was. All I could get out was 10. Tommy came and found me and I wept, saying, "It's a 14. My pain level is 14. Endone isn't working. I need something else."

It felt as if the Endone was going straight to my head. My eyes felt puffy and blurry and I felt woozy, but the pain would not ease up at all. Finally, they gave me more medication and it started to subside. To say I was off my head is an understatement. Charlie had been transferred to NICU and put on C-PAP as he was having some difficulty breathing. Tommy returned to NICU and Facetimed me so I could see him.

"Oh, is that a dog in his room? How cute!" I said.

"Babe, there is definitely not a dog in NICU…"

Yeah, haha. I was cooked.

EPILOGUE

Our NICU journey with Charlie was much smoother than the journey with Harry. We still experienced the odd hiccup or two, when Charlie had a collapsed lung on Day 2 and needed to be ventilated, along with a chest tube. But being back in this hospital meant our trust in the team was so deep that we didn't have any concerns whatsoever. We knew that we could relax and our baby was in the best hands. It was quite healing for me to be back in this NICU; almost as though a loop got to be closed. We had spent a huge chunk of time in these hallways, seeing the faces of the wonderful staff, and the impact it had on both Tommy and me was quite moving. What we hadn't banked on was the impact we had had on the staff. Obviously, we were excited to be back; but having the nurses and doctors light up and run to give us a hug, and visibly excited to have us, was quite a shock. But not in a bad way. I hadn't ever stopped to think that perhaps we'd had any sort of effect on people from the time we'd spent here with Harry. It was beautiful, and it felt like home.

During my pregnancy with Charlie, I had opted to stay medicated. Working with my psychiatrist, I had shifted from Sertraline, which kept wearing off, to a different drug called Pristiq, or Desvenlefexine. This was 100% my jam. I hadn't had any issues with it wearing off and was able to halve my dose throughout pregnancy. The benefit to me and my mental health outweighed the potential risks the medication had to the baby. My postpartum journey with Charlie was vastly different to my experiences with Addie and Harry; the main difference was that I didn't experience that huge postpartum hormonal dump that made me feel like a lunatic. I just felt level. Clearly, my mental health was noticeable to the NICU staff. I had so many of them say how much better I looked this time around, and I had no problems blurting out, "Yeah it's because I'm medicated!" I couldn't stop telling everyone how amazing it was to be medicated and not feel as out of control as I had with Harry.

I had my postpartum check up with a midwife who had previously looked after me with Harry. She was lovely, and quite impressed at how level and calm I appeared to be, despite having a 31-weeker in NICU with a collapsed lung and chest drain on a ventilator. I explained to her that I was medicated and it was the best thing I'd ever done. We ended up talking further about medication and after she opened up to me about her first postpartum experience and the intrusive thoughts she experienced along with severe anxiety, I couldn't stress to her enough how much I recommended that she stay on her medication if she decided to have another baby. I am not someone who would usually advocate for medication; I'm all for the natural route on just about everything. But having experienced postpartum twice unmedicated and once medicated, I fully believe that the way every woman is expected to navigate the biggest hormonal and chemical imbalance a human being can possibly go through, all whilst trying to heal and care for their baby, is almost inhumane. There needs to be some sort of high dose natural supplement you can take postpartum that helps mothers adjust, rather than us having to raw-dog our way through pure irrationality. And look, maybe there is something like this available and I just didn't do enough research. I sure hope there is, because there certainly is a need for it.

The slogan for our time in this hospital soon became *Stay medicated!* and the nurses and doctors alike were joining in on the banter.

EPILOGUE

That's what I loved about this place. It felt like you were dealing with friends and was such a warm environment in which to have your baby cared for. Charlie and I were discharged from this hospital at bang on 36 weeks gestation and rather than going via RFDS, we opted to drive home. My lovely mother was the chauffeur as Tommy was now back home with Addie and Harry. We arrived home late, and it was a great feeling to bring Charlie into our house. Addie woke up the next morning not knowing that we'd returned and as soon as she saw me, she ran to me and wanted to hold her baby Charlie. She was, and still is, a beautiful big sister.

When writing this epilogue, I first reread the previous chapter and couldn't believe what I had written in terms of wishing for a baby that would just fit into the chaos and didn't require so much of me. That is exactly what we got with Charlie. He was a calm, contented little newborn and I was able to successfully breastfeed him for nine months. We only stopped because he started using my nipple as a chew toy. This little boy brought so much healing for me and made me see what so many people talk about when they say they love the newborn stage. Along with healing, it also brought some sadness; it made me sad that I had been so unwell for Addie and Harry, that I missed out on enjoying being a mum for the longest time. It made me sad that I hadn't given Addie and Harry this medicated version of me, and I wondered whether, if I had been medicated, the journey might have been different. Would I have been able to breastfeed? Would I have been able to deal with the challenges differently? So many questions I will never get answers to.

What I do know is that Charlie was sent to me for a reason. As I've said in previous chapters, I was meant to be Addie and Harry's mum; there is no doubt about that. But I think I somehow manifested Charlie into this world to complete our little puzzle and heal the many broken parts of me. As of right now, I am still on the same dose of medication as when I was pregnant. I am proud that I have never had to increase the dosage. Don't get me wrong – there have been plenty of times when I've thought I needed to! But I have come to realise that it is okay to feel overwhelmed as a mother. It is okay for your kids to see you completely lose your shit, because they need to see that you are human. What is more important is showing them how you recover from the outburst, how you apologise and explain how you got to that point.

I spent so much time trying to be the perfect parent who never got angry out of fear it would damage my children, only to realise I was damaging myself in the process. Every human being on the planet gets angry, and if we don't show our children what anger or frustration looks like, how are they meant to survive in the world? How are they meant to understand it if one day their boss gets angry, or a client of theirs gets angry at them? It is so unrealistic. Parents today face a lot of pressure with social media playing on all of our anxieties and insecurities. If you yell one time, you are soon faced with advertisements on how to complete a course and stop being a yelling parent. It's bullshit. I don't know what the answer is here. All I know is that I choose to continually work on bettering myself and growing with my children and the world around us so that we can all try to exist in an ever-changing environment. Anyway, enough about my philosophies on parenting.

The whole point of this epilogue is to highlight that my mental health is still a work in progress, and I believe it always will be.

EPILOGUE

I survived postpartum for the third time, for the most part unscathed, and Charlie has fitted into our chaotic world perfectly. In November 2022, my mother and I started delivering antenatal workshops to expecting parents in our local area, and we have dedicated a section to postpartum depression and anxiety, which Tommy and I present. The feedback we have received has been fantastic, especially from the partner's point of view. Our intention is not to scare people, but to highlight how scary things can get. Obviously, mine was a severe case; but I talk to many women who feel comfortable enough to talk to me about the intrusive thoughts they have had once they had a baby. Things from as simple as "maybe I'm a bad mum because I don't want to pick her up right now" to going for a walk by a river and thinking "what if I just threw him in the water". These are very real intrusive thoughts that occur, and it happens to the best of us.

If nothing else, I want this book to start conversations between partners and potentially start a greater conversation during postpartum check-ups. I want this book to help people realise they aren't crazy for having intense and sometimes violent thoughts. Women need to feel comfortable enough to talk about these things without fear of judgment or being deemed unfit to be a parent. It can be terrifying. Throw in lack of sleep, an assault on all your senses, and the overwhelming love or protection you feel for this tiny little person, and it can make you feel like a lunatic. It can also be extremely hard for partners to comprehend, through no fault of their own. My only advice is to talk about it. Say it out loud, no matter how scary the thought is. Don't stop talking about it.

I have said before how alone I felt in my journey, despite having all the support and love in the world. I believe that it was because very few people ever talked about their own intrusive thoughts... Or perhaps they just didn't experience them as I did? Who knows. What I do know is that the idea of another woman feeling so alone and afraid of her own mind breaks my heart. At the end of every antenatal course, I offer people the opportunity to reach out to me postpartum if they need to. I have had this offer taken up, and I dropped everything to meet with the mother and simply listen. What a profound impact that had on her journey! It's something she will probably never forget. I didn't do it to be able to write about it; I did it in the hope that I could help her to never feel alone and scared and misunderstood. I would do it for anyone.

Since we had Charlie, Tommy has had the snip, so we are officially at the end of our story with bringing little people into the world. I couldn't be happier with our little trio of ratbags. They test me in ways that I can't even explain, but more importantly, they fill me with pride and bring great joy and love to our household. To have all three of them earthside, I wouldn't change a thing.

Printed in the USA
CPSIA information can be obtained
at www.ICGtesting.com
CBHW030803230724
11983CB00022B/92